THE CONFESSIONS OF ANTHONY FAUCI

THE CONFESSIONS OF ANTHONY FAUCI

ROBERT KENNEDY III

MAHA
BOOKS

MAHA Books may be purchased in bulk at special discounts for sales promotion, corporate gifts, fund-raising, or educational purposes. Special editions can also be created to specifications. For details, contact the Special Sales Department, Skyhorse Publishing, 307 West 36th Street, 11th Floor, New York, NY 10018 or info@skyhorsepublishing.com.

MAHA Books® and Skyhorse Publishing® are registered trademarks of Skyhorse Publishing, Inc.®, a Delaware corporation.

Visit our website at www.skyhorsepublishing.com.
Please follow our publisher Tony Lyons on Instagram @tonylyonsisuncertain.

10 9 8 7 6 5 4 3 2 1

Library of Congress Cataloging-in-Publication Data is available on file.

Hardcover ISBN: 978-1-63144-086-1
Ebook ISBN: 978-1-63144-087-8

Cover design by Brian Peterson
Book design by Geoff Towle

Printed in the United States of America

Contents

On January 20, 2025, just a few hours before leaving office, President Joe Biden issued a preemptive pardon for Anthony Fauci, removing any possible penalties for any known or unknown criminal offenses against the United States dating back to January 1, 2014.

Executive Grant of Clemency

JOSEPH R. BIDEN, JR.
President of the United States of America

TO ALL TO WHOM THESE PRESENTS SHALL COME, GREETING:

BE IT KNOWN, THAT THIS DAY, I, JOSEPH R. BIDEN, JR., PRESIDENT OF THE UNITED STATES, PURSUANT TO MY POWERS UNDER ARTICLE II, SECTION 2, CLAUSE 1, OF THE CONSTITUTION, HAVE GRANTED UNTO

DR. ANTHONY S. FAUCI

A FULL AND UNCONDITIONAL PARDON

FOR ANY OFFENSES against the United States which he may have committed or taken part in during the period from January 1, 2014, through the date of this pardon arising from or in any manner related to his service as Director of the National Institute of Allergy and Infectious Diseases, as a member of the White House Coronavirus Task Force or the White House COVID-19 Response Team, or as Chief Medical Advisor to the President.

IN TESTIMONY WHEREOF I have hereunto signed my name and caused the seal of the Department of Justice to be affixed.

Done at the City of Washington this 19th day of January in the year of our Lord Two Thousand and Twenty-Five and of the Independence of the United States the Two Hundred and Forty-Ninth.

JOSEPH R. BIDEN, JR.
President

A NOTE TO THE READER

Let Me Be Perfectly Clear...

They told me I'd never write this.

They told me I *shouldn't* write this.

But when your name is on a half-billion in grants, your fingerprints are in every virus freezer from Galveston to Guangdong, and Congress suddenly develops a spine—it's not a question of *if* the subpoenas come. It's a question of how loud they echo.

So let's get one thing straight, right up front:

If I did anything wrong —*IF*— then everybody else was doing it too.

You think I'm being evasive? I *was* the highest-paid employee in the federal government for twenty years. Evasion is the job. They're saying I funded the creation of a pandemic.

We were in the middle of a *biodefense boom.* The Pentagon was flinging money at anything that could breathe and mutate. You think I'm going to turn that down? Please. I had a budget bigger than thirty countries' militaries. I was doing 3D chess while the CDC was still learning Connect Four.

So when Peter Daszak came in, eyes lit up, babbling about bats, spike proteins, and "Disease X," I didn't ask *too many* questions. That's not what NIAID does. We disburse. We nod. We reauthorize.

And yes, I told Congress *we didn't* fund gain-of-function in Wuhan. Because we didn't. Not by **our** definition.

You want to know the real kicker? We thought we were the smart ones. We thought we had the Chinese on a leash.
Turns out, we were holding the leash, but someone else had the collar.

Look, maybe it wasn't smart to outsource the most dangerous biological research in the world to a half-inspected BSL-4 facility run by a military dictatorship. Maybe it wasn't smart to send money through a zoologist named Peter who did podcast interviews like he was starring in *Contagion 2: The Reckoning*. But that's how science works. You juggle pathogens and pray the budget gets renewed.

Now the subpoenas are flying.
They've got email threads, contracts, DEFUSE proposals, and a photo of me at the Milken Institute talking about how a good pandemic could "blow up the system." (That was metaphorical. Mostly.)

And suddenly everyone's pretending they didn't sign off on this.
The Pentagon, the White House, the NSC, the WHO.
Even the CIA's pretending they weren't involved. (Cute.)

I know how this works. I've testified under oath more times than half the Judiciary Committee has been sober.
I wasn't willing to go down with the entire virology complex without a fat advance on the backend and a Bolivian passport in my sock. Or maybe a Presidential pardon.

Am I saying I am above the law?

Above, below, adjacent—doesn't really apply. With the highest national security clearance, with the military and intelligence communities being my neighborhoods, we never thought about getting into trouble. We created trouble.

And then rescued everyone.

So yeah, I'm writing this book.
Not because I want to. Because I have to.
Because the truth is coming out anyway.
And I'd rather be the one telling it.

—AF

INTRODUCTION
Just the Facts

I didn't plan to tell you everything.

That was never the deal.

The whole point was: I protect the system, the system protects me.
I carry the water, I keep the secrets, and in return?
I get to leave on my own terms. Retire.
Disappear.
Take a few board seats. Write a carefully curated memoir. Maybe get a Netflix doc.

But the moment they floated *immunity* in a hearing?

The moment my own people started distancing themselves?

The deal was off.

So fine.

You want the truth?

Here it is.

Yes—we funded research that made viruses more dangerous.
Yes—we pushed that research offshore so we wouldn't get caught in our own jurisdiction.
Yes—we used EcoHealth as a cutout.
Yes—we knew Wuhan's BSL-4 was a joke.
Yes—we saw signs something leaked in 2019 and still said nothing.
Yes—we lied about masks.
Yes—we moved the vaccine goalposts because we were afraid of panic. Yes—we censored dissent because we didn't trust you to think critically. Yes—we called things misinformation *before we knew if they were true or not.*

And no—none of that was by accident.

You want to know why?

Because **we thought we were the adults in the room**.

We thought if we let the public into the conversation, they'd blow up our labs and hang us from lampposts.

We thought *you* were the risk—not the virus.

So we shaped the story.
We told half-truths.
We rigged the peer review process.
We buried early treatment data that didn't fit the narrative.
We locked down healthy children and called it "mitigation."

And every time we crossed a line,
we told ourselves it was **for the greater good**.

But the truth?

It wasn't about health.

It was about control.

It was about saving institutions, not lives.

It was about **keeping the whole fragile apparatus from tipping over**—funding, reputation, liability, diplomacy, legacy.

We thought if we just held it together long enough, we could rewrite the ending.

That maybe history would forgive us if we delivered a miracle.

But history doesn't care about motives.

Only consequences.

And now?

The consequences are coming. So yeah.

I'm talking now.

Not because I want to.

But because I already know **what happens if I don't**.

If I did most of what people think I did —and I did— the pardon means I can stop pretending otherwise.

No more spin.
No more denials.

Just the facts.

Unpleasant.
Unredacted.
And overdue.

CHAPTER 1

The Game (and How to Play It)

I'm not going to tell you everything in this chapter.
Not because I can't.
Because I won't.
Not yet.

There's a rhythm to this.
You don't open with the whole crime.
You lay down the **harmless parts**, let people feel smart for noticing the cracks, and then—when they think they've caught up—you drop the real thing.

That's how I've always done it.

Omission isn't lying.
It's… professional discretion.
A survival skill.

If I told you everything up front, you'd either shut the book or burn it.
But my job here is to keep you turning pages.
Curiosity beats conscience every time.

So here's what I will say:

This didn't start in Wuhan.
Not in a market.
Not in a lab.

Where it really started was Geneva.
1975.
The **Biological Weapons Convention**.

We said the right things back then.
We always do.
No more engineered plagues. No more state-sponsored pathogens.

We outlawed the weapon—**but not the research**.

That was the loophole.
That's always the loophole.

You can't develop bioweapons.
But you *can* study potential "pandemic agents."
You can't build offensive viruses.
But you *can* build them for "defensive purposes"—as long as you say it's to prepare.

So we kept the science alive.
Just changed the labels.
"Gain-of-function" became "predictive modeling."
"Weaponization" became "public health readiness."

Same virus. Different pitch.

And we told ourselves it was fine because we'd buried the intent under enough layers of ethics committees and PowerPoint slides.

But the infrastructure?
It stayed.

It all started in a **treaty we never really honored.**
The **Biological Weapons Convention**—1975, Geneva—was supposed to be the firewall.
It banned development, production, and stockpiling of biological weapons.
Full stop.
But here's the quiet part no one says aloud:
It had no enforcement mechanism.
No inspection regime.
No audit trail.
No consequences.

It was an honor system for nations that don't operate on honor.

The U.S. signed it. So did Russia. So did China.

And then?

We built **an entire bioweapons infrastructure** inside the margins.

Not with bombs or missiles.
With grants.

We used **biodefense funding** as the backdoor.
After 9/11 and the anthrax letters, that door blew off its hinges.

Suddenly, we weren't just researching pathogens—we were **enhancing them**.
To "understand how they might evolve."
To "prepare for worst-case scenarios."
To "defend against hypothetical attacks."

But functionally?

We were doing **everything BWC was designed to prevent**.

Creating novel viruses.
Tinkering with zoonotic jump potential.
Mapping out the exact mutations that would make a pathogen *unstoppable*.

And not in secret, either.

We called it **gain-of-function research**.
We published it.
We funded it through NIH, NIAID, BARDA, DARPA.
We subcontracted it through EcoHealth to labs like WIV.

And we stamped "public health" on every page.

Here's the trick:

The BWC only bans *weapons*.
But a virus in a freezer isn't a weapon—until it's **deployed**.

So we said, "This isn't a weapon.
It's a study. A countermeasure. A simulation."

It's not **weaponization**, we told ourselves.
It's **understanding the threat landscape**.

And when you put that in a grant application?

It clears.

Every time.

So no, this didn't start in a market.
Or even a lab.
It started in a legal framework that **looked like a safeguard** but **functioned as a green light**.

We banned the thing.
Then we renamed it.

And from there?
All we had to do was call it *science.*

Let me just say it plainly now—because someone has to:
Creating the next pandemic in the lab doesn't help you stop the next pandemic.

It just makes it more likely **you'll start one**.

We called it preparedness.
We said we needed to "get ahead" of what nature might do.
So we built viruses that nature hadn't built yet.

Think about that.

We were playing with loaded weapons—then telling Congress we were "stress-testing the system."

That's not science.
That's a **controlled demolition** with no evacuation plan.

Here's why it doesn't hold up—scientifically, strategically, or even statistically:

1. **There are millions of potential zoonotic viruses.**
   We don't even have names for most of them.
   The chance that the one we build in a lab is the exact one nature cooks up next?
   Astronomically small. Laughable.
2. **There are infinite mutation pathways.**
   You can tweak spike proteins all day, but the odds of matching natural evolution—right mutation, right receptor, right species jump—are practically zero.
3. **Even if we "guessed right"... so what?**
   There's no infrastructure to mass-produce and distribute vaccines *before* the pandemic starts.

You don't pre-vaccinate 8 billion people for a virus that doesn't exist.
By the time you need the vaccine, **it's too late**.

That's not defense.
That's playing with matches **in a fireworks factory**.

And we knew this.

But we said it anyway.

Because it **sounded smart**.
It made the work sound noble.
And more importantly—it **kept the funding flowing**.

Pandemic prevention is a gold mine.
Every government wants it.
Every lab wants a slice.
Every defense agency wants to show it can control the uncontrollable.

So we lied.

Not by saying the viruses were safe.
But by pretending the research was useful.

You don't stop bioterror by showing everyone how to build better bioweapons.
You don't protect the village by breeding the dragon.
You don't "study evolution" by *forcing it.*

This wasn't preparation.
It was provocation.

If I told you I was preventing arson by **designing new kinds of gasoline**, you'd laugh.

If I said I was working to stop future train derailments by **building more unstable trains**, you'd call the cops.

But if I say we're enhancing bat coronaviruses with human ACE2 binding to **"model potential spillover events"**?

Suddenly it's visionary.

I did what I did in a system that mistook **building bombs** for **writing instruction manuals**.

And when it blew up?

We pretended it was a **natural disaster**.

Because the alternative?

Was admitting we were the architects.

Look—
It wasn't my fault.
And I'll tell you why.

This whole thing?
This idea that *I* created the system, that *I* designed the monster—
Wrong.

I was handed the machine.

The gears were already turning.
The money was already flowing.
The labs were already pitching chimeric viruses like they were reality show pilots.

When I got the keys, it wasn't "Should we do this?"
It was:
"Which variant are we funding next?"

You want to blame me for building the virus?

Fine.
But first blame the **treaties we never enforced**.
Then blame the **generals who wanted bio-deterrence on the cheap**.
Then blame the **universities that chased gain-of-function grants like lottery tickets**.

By the time I showed up with the checkbook, the virology world was already a casino. I didn't invent the game.
I just **learned to play it really well**.

CHAPTER 2

The Rule We Don't Say Out Loud

Because If You Say It, You Have to Admit What Game You're In

You want to know the rule?

The real rule?

It's not in any NIH charter.
It's not in the P3CO guidance.

It's definitely not in the Biological Weapons Convention.

But it governs everything.

And we all knew it.

You don't build a virus like that unless you want someone to see it.

You don't share samples unless you want someone to know **you have more**.

And you don't send it to China unless you're sending a message.

The message?

"We can do it too."

This was never about vaccines.
It was about **positioning**.

Deterrence.
Parity.
Signaling.

You want to know what PREDICT was?

It wasn't a surveillance program.

It was a **delivery mechanism for showing our hand—without showing the whole deck**.

We didn't hand them the blueprint for the apocalypse.
We handed them **just enough** to remind them what we were capable of.

It's not collaboration.
It's **controlled exposure**.

Same doctrine we used in the Cold War—
only this time, it's not missiles in silos.

It's sequences in freezers.

Why else would we risk it?

Why else ship samples to a lab known to blur the line between academic and military research?

Why else tolerate a place like WIV if not to use it?

We weren't naive.

We weren't sloppy.

We were operating under **a doctrine that doesn't have a name** but functions like religion:

If they can do it, we have to show we can do it too—faster, cleaner, better.

And if we can't stop them, we make sure they know what happens if they try anything stupid.

That's not health diplomacy.

That's **Mutually Assured Contagion**.

No one wanted to say it.
Because the moment you name it, you admit what you're actually doing.

You're not preparing for pandemics.
You're building **the threat landscape**—then calling it defense.

You're designing what you hope **never gets used**
and building it **just in case it does**.

And that's the real virus.

Not the one that spreads by breath.

The one that spreads by **justification**.

I acted inside a system that already decided **some viruses aren't built to stop pandemics**.

They're built so the other side doesn't start one.

And we all agreed—

We'd never say that out loud.

Until now.

CHAPTER 3

The Bat Cave Boys

How a Wildlife NGO Became DARPA's Favorite Laundromat

If you want to move money without people noticing, you don't go through Lockheed. You go through something soft. Something green.

See, after the Obama-era gain-of-function moratorium, we all had to get a little creative.
The Pandemic Pathogen Care and Oversight (P3CO) framework was the illusion of oversight.
No project was ever rejected under it—not because they were all safe, but because the people submitting the proposals were also the ones deciding what "gain-of-function" meant.

It's like asking the getaway driver if what he's doing is technically illegal, while handing him the map.

But he understood the game. He knew the lingo.

He knew that if you promised "spillover surveillance," you could get funded for **predictive pandemic modeling, gain-of-**

function recombination studies, and the occasional "synthetic recombinant infectious clone" tucked discreetly into the supplementary materials.

What did he call it?
Ah yes—**"risk of emergence"** research.
In other words: "Let's build it and see if it could happen."

I don't remember who said "build the bomb to understand how someone *might* build the bomb," but Peter made it a business model.

Now let's talk **DEFUSE**.

Peter's 2018 proposal to DARPA was bold.
Too bold.
Insert furin cleavage sites into SARS-like viruses to see if you can make them more infectious in humans.
Release aerosolized nanoparticles in bat caves to deliver recombinant vaccines.
Oh, and do it in partnership with the Wuhan Institute of Virology, because of course.

DARPA said no.
But NIH didn't.

At least, **not on paper**.

DEFUSE wasn't a research proposal.

It was ***a schematic for deniability***.

The kind you write when you already know the thing you're describing **either already exists** or is being quietly built across three continents.

You've heard of it by now—maybe.

If you haven't?

Let me ruin your evening.

September 2018.
DARPA receives a proposal.

From who?

EcoHealth Alliance.
On behalf of **Wuhan Institute of Virology, UNC**, and a few other familiar faces. The title?

"Project DEFUSE: Defusing the Threat of
Bat-Borne Coronaviruses."

Sounds friendly.

Sounds preventative.

Sounds like ***exactly what you'd say if you were planning to build something no treaty would let you fund publicly***.

It laid out the whole thing:

- Insert ***furin cleavage sites*** into bat SARS-like viruses
- Use ***barcoded recombinants*** for tracking
- Pass them through ***humanized mice***
- Hide the research behind ***"conservation goals"***

- Coordinate sample transfers through ***field partners in Asia***

We're not talking "modeling" here.

We're talking ***full-chain construction of pandemic-class viruses*** that could cross the human-animal barrier, evade immune systems, and ***be tracked post-release***.

Just in case, right?

Sure.

DARPA rejected it.
Officially.

Said it was ***too risky***.

Which is a nice way of saying:

"We'd love to do this but we don't want to get caught funding it directly."

So what happened?

It got done anyway.

Some of it at UNC.
Some of it at WIV.
And some of it—this is where it gets spicy—through ***Metabiota***.

Metabiota, for those just joining the party, is a so-called "pandemic risk modeling company."

They received ***millions from USAID*** to collect, store, and ship pathogen samples around the globe.

Also: **Hunter Biden's firm Rosemont Seneca invested in them**.

Yes. That Hunter.

No, not by accident.

And yes—there were ***emails***.

Emails about Metabiota's "strategic value" in Ukraine.
Emails about their **alignment with EcoHealth**.
Emails with Peter Daszak's name not far behind.

All in ***Hunter's inbox***.

Which makes things awkward when ***you're trying to explain why Metabiota was routing avian flu and coronavirus samples through China*** while sitting on the Biden cap table.

But don't worry.

They ***made it disappear***.

DEFUSE was the project that told you ***what was coming***.

The laptop was the one that told you ***who helped build it***.

And the pardon?

That was the ***receipt***.

No trial.
No headlines.
Just ***the pen signing itself***.

Like everything else in this story—

It looked automated.

But someone still built the program.

The Proposal Wasn't About COVID

Everyone thinks DEFUSE was about **SARS-CoV-2.**

Wrong.

DEFUSE was about ***proving you could build one like it—and hide the fingerprints.***

COVID was just the first strain to hit public servers.

The real play?

Build ***the method.***

Look at the language.

It doesn't say "develop countermeasures."

It says:

"Identify, characterize, and manipulate high-risk zoonotic viruses with pandemic potential."

Big difference.

One is defense.

The other is ***inventory.***

Here's the real genius of it:

They proposed inserting **furin cleavage sites** into SARS-like bat viruses—

not because those mutations were expected—

but because they ***weren't***.

Quote:

"…furin sites are not found in these viruses naturally, and their presence may enhance pathogenicity."

Which means:

"If we add one and it breaks out, no one can say it came from nature—except us."

That's not a red flag.

That's a ***pre-installed cover story***.

They proposed ***barcoded virus libraries*** so they could ***track which synthetic versions spread fastest in animal models***.

That's gain-of-function with ***analytics baked in***.

That's not a health project.

That's ***beta testing***.

They planned to do it in ***China, Laos, and other "hot zones,"*** not because it was safer—

but because ***regulatory oversight was looser***.

So was accountability.

And shipping.

(Ask Metabiota.)

And when DARPA said “No”?

They didn’t say “Stop.”

They said:

“This exceeds acceptable risk under the current USG framework.”

Translation:

“Not under our name.”

So they routed it through ***EcoHealth***.

Let ***Wuhan*** run the wet work.
Let ***DTRA*** run the modeling.
Let ***Metabiota*** handle the shipping.
Let ***UC Davis*** pretend to look surprised.

And what did I do?

I ***kept the money flowing***.

Quietly.
Cleanly.
Without direct fingerprints.

Because DEFUSE didn't need approval.

It just needed ***deniability***.

DEFUSE wasn't a virus plan.

It was a ***virus business model***.

Build the strain.
Study the chaos.
Sell the solution.
Hide the receipt.

And when it leaks?

Blame the bat.

The Architects Never Leave the Building

You want to know how you spot a covert op in a lab coat?

The same three names keep showing up—
and ***none of them ever go away***.

No firings.
No hearings.
No public disgrace.

Just ***more grants***.

And ***book deals***.

Start with ***Peter Daszak***.

DEFUSE's mouthpiece.
EcoHealth's guilt sponge.
Part-time "conservationist," full-time ***cutout***.

He didn't write the code.
He didn't clone the inserts.
But he ***signed the grant***.
And ***laundered the risk***.

When DEFUSE got too hot?

He ***pivoted to narrative management***.

Wrote the ***Lancet letter***.
Corralled "27 scientists" to say lab leak was a ***conspiracy***.
Didn't mention he wrote the damn thing.

That's not science.

That's ***containment***.

Then there's ***Ralph Baric***.

The architect.
Quiet. Clean. Surgical.

Baric doesn't do headlines.
He does ***templates***.

His lab built ***chimeric SARS backbones*** before DEFUSE was even drafted.

He warned us—
then built it anyway.

That's the trick.

Do the research.
Then publish the warning.

It's ***a liability shield.***
And it works.

Ask him how many times he's testified under oath.

Spoiler: ***Zero.***

And of course, ***Shi Zhengli.***
The "Bat Woman."

She was ***already running DEFUSE-adjacent work*** when the proposal landed.

She didn't need permission.

She needed ***material.***
And ***Metabiota*** made sure she had it.

You think we didn't know?

We ***helped*** her do it.

Not directly. Not in an email.

But through ***funding paths*** and ***winks.***

These weren't rogue actors.

They were ***strategic assets***.

Each with a lane.

- Daszak ran cover.
- Baric built blueprints.
- Shi ran the factory.
- I handled ***continuity***.

The Rejection Was the Green Light

People love to say:

"Well, DARPA rejected DEFUSE. So it never happened."

Right.

And I guess if you unplug a smoke detector, it means there's no fire either.

Let me explain something about ***rejections*** in D.C.:

They're not denials.
They're ***absolution***.

DARPA's official response?

"This work does not fall within the scope of current USG gain-of-function policies. The risks are deemed excessive given the potential outcomes and current safeguards."

Sounds responsible, right?

Reads like ***a firewall***.

And that's exactly what it was.

A ***paper shield***.

So when something went wrong later?

They could say:

"Wasn't us. We said no."

Meanwhile?

The **network** went active.

Because saying no isn't the same as ***stopping it***.

They didn't alert Congress.
Didn't alert NIH.
Didn't freeze EcoHealth funding.
Didn't warn international partners.

You know what they did?

Nothing.

They rejected it **knowing** the people involved would keep going.

And knowing ***we'd let them***.

You know how I know?

Because two months after the rejection, ***funding continued***.

Through **USAID**.
Through **NIH subgrants**.
Through **Metabiota**.
Through **DTRA**.
Through ***the usual paths***.

The only thing that stopped was ***the visibility***.

That's how biowarfare works in the 21st century.

You don't need a secret base.

You need ***distributed plausible deniability***.

Put the researchers in one country.
Put the samples in another.
Put the money through a third.
And put the blame on ***nature***.

And when the proposal leaks—like it eventually did?

You get to say:

"It was never approved."

And that's technically true.

But ***practically meaningless***.

Because **rejection was the signal**.

The wink.

The nod.

The "you're on your own now—but we won't stop you."

And they didn't.

And we didn't.

And I didn't...

It didn't happen through approval.

It was through ***architecture***.

I built a system where saying "no" was ***safer than saying yes*** — and ***meant the same thing anyway***.

The Samples Had Passports

You want to understand DEFUSE?

Forget the proposals.

Follow the ***samples***.

They don't talk about this much.

Because once you start tracking the viruses—not the papers, not the press releases, but the ***actual vials***—

you start noticing something:

They all know each other.

Like cousins.

Same binding domains.
Same backbones.
Same ***serial numbers, sometimes***.

That's not zoonosis.

That's ***supply chain***.

Start in ***Yunnan, China***.

Bat caves.
Rural outposts.
Metabiota field teams with coolers and gloves.

They collect ***hundreds of samples***.

From bats, birds, pigs, civets, pangolins, dirt, whatever moves.

Send them to ***Wuhan***.

Label them: "SARS-like," "AIV-like," "unknown recombinants."

Now you split the tree.

Some go to:

- **WIV** – for gain-of-function and transfection modeling
- **UNC** – for recombinant chimera construction
- **USAMRIID** – for "defensive study"
- **Duke-NUS** – for immune escape research
- **UC Davis** – for database storage and mapping

Same samples.
Different "use cases."

All with ***quiet agreements*** not to share full results with each other.

Why?

So no one ***knows everything***.

Classic compartmentalization.

Old CIA move. Still works.

But here's the kicker.

Those same ***recombinant fragments***?

Show up **again** in SARS-CoV-2's genome.

And in ***avian flu strains*** that "shouldn't have those insertions."

And in ***retracted preprints*** that nobody wants to explain.

Over and over.

Like ***a lab accidentally photocopying its own crime scene***.

You don't get furin sites in that configuration by chance.

You don't get ***codon optimization to human expression*** from a wet market.

You don't get ***novel spike-RBD combinations*** with ***barcoding systems embedded*** unless ***someone's tracking the behavior***.

And we were.

We always were.

So when people say:

"There's no proof this came from DEFUSE."

I nod.

Because ***technically, they're right***.

You won't find a barcode that says "Property of Peter Daszak."

But if you trace the samples?

You'll find ***DEFUSE fingerprints on every glass slide in the outbreak chain***.

Not all at once.

But ***enough to recognize the pattern***.

It wasn't a single virus.

It was a ***network of viruses—***

collected, modified, shipped, and sequenced
like ***global inventory***.

And like any good logistics system—

it only leaks when ***someone forgets to relabel the box***.

It Wasn't a Virus, It Was a Version Tree

Here's what people still get wrong:

DEFUSE wasn't about engineering ***one virus***.

It was about ***engineering all of them***.

Or at least ***a library***—
each with a ***different failure point***.

Think software testing.

You don't run one program and pray it works.

You fork it.

You change a line.
Test the result.
Record the behavior.
Repeat.

That's what DEFUSE was.

A ***live mutation workshop***.

- Insert furin site? See what happens.
- Change codons? Track expression speed.
- Add humanized receptor binding? Count transmission.
- Spike protein swap? Measure immune escape.

Each "virus" wasn't a threat.

It was ***a data point***.

And where did they test this?

Ferrets.
Humanized mice.
Cell lines.

They weren't just watching for ***pathogenicity***.

They were watching for ***performance***.

Not "Is it lethal?"

But ***"Does it scale?"***

That's what people miss about gain-of-function.

It's not always about building the **deadliest virus**.

It's about building the ***most reliable platform***.

Something that can be ***controlled, tracked, adjusted***.

And if it leaks?

You already know ***how it behaves***.

DEFUSE wasn't the crime.

It was the ***planning phase***.

The whiteboard.
The Gantt chart.
The virus family tree, with ***notes in the margins***.

And somewhere on that tree?

The ***exact version*** that became SARS-CoV-2.

Maybe not on purpose.

Maybe not by mistake.

Maybe just ***ahead of schedule***.

No-See-Um Seams

Let's talk about Baric.

Not the man.

The method.

"No-see-um."

Sounds cute, right?

Like a mosquito you can't swat.

But what it really meant?

Genomic laundering.

Most synthetic viruses leave scars.

Restriction sites.
Cloning markers.
Codon weirdness.
Stitch lines you can spot if you know what to look for.

So Baric—being Baric—asked:

“What if we could hide the surgery?”

That’s what no-see-um was.

Not a new tool.

A new ***invisibility cloak***.

It worked like this:

You break the viral genome into fragments.
Engineer them separately.
Then reassemble using **seamless ligation**—enzymatic techniques that **don’t leave scars**.

No restriction enzyme footprints.
No ligation signatures.

Result?

A virus that looks like it came out of nature.

Except it didn’t.

It came out of ***North Carolina***.

And for years?

It worked.

No-see-um let us build chimeric viruses, recombinant backbones, codon-optimized monsters—

with no telltale signs.

You sequence it?

It looks clean.

You analyze it?

It looks plausible.

Even I'll admit: it was ***a masterpiece of denial engineering***.

But here's the punchline.

It left a mark anyway.

Not a cut. A ***pattern***.

Because when you write code—even genomic code—
you leave a ***style***.

And Baric's style?

It showed up in SARS-CoV-2.

In the **codon choices**.
In the **rare synonymous substitutions**.
In the ***restriction site spacing***.

Tiny anomalies.

Nothing you'd notice at first glance.

But forensic virologists?

They noticed.

Bruttel, Washburne, Segreto.

They looked.

And they ***saw it***.

The genome wasn't seamless.

It was ***too perfect***.

Too optimized.
Too conveniently cuttable.
Too close to ***Baric's published ligation map***.

That's not nature.

That's ***the ghost of the lab coat***.

I didn't hide the evidence.

Baric did.

And then ***his technique leaked through the seams***.

Like a watermark on a classified file.

Like ***a name whispered in the code***.

Unprovable Means Untouchable

The beauty of no-see-um?

Wasn't just that it fooled scientists.

It fooled ***lawyers***.

And that's what really mattered.

We weren't trying to convince a virologist.

We were trying to ***beat the burden of proof***.

Because once you remove the seams, the cuts, the flags—you remove ***intent***.

And if you remove intent?

You remove ***liability***.

Think about it:

What do you need to prove a lab origin?

A footprint.
A marker.
A traceable construct.
A one-to-one match with a known recombinant template.

No-see-um deleted the breadcrumbs.

It made the virus ***plausibly deniable***.

Which meant:

- No FOIA risk.
- No congressional subpoena trail.
- No grant suspension.
- No jail time.

- No headlines.
- No ***accountability***.

And that's why we loved it.

Not because it made better viruses.

Because it made ***smoother crimes***.

If something leaked?

We could shrug.

"It looks natural."

"We've seen this in bats before."

"Sure, the furin site's odd—but nothing we can prove."

We didn't have to lie.

We just had to **leave out what couldn't be seen**.

And Baric gave us ***exactly that***.

But here's the part you might not get:

The ***method*** was more powerful than the virus.

Because it became **policy**.

A firewall.

A ***shield for the entire program***.

As long as we used no-see-um:

- The edits were invisible
- The inserts were seamless
- The genome was clean
- The chain of custody didn't matter

Even if it leaked.

Even if it spread.

Even if millions died.

If the sequence ***looked natural***?

We ***walked away clean***.

Until someone noticed the pattern.

Until ***Bruttel cracked the code***.

Until the method ***left a scar it was never supposed to***.

Because the only thing worse than a crime?

A crime that tries too hard to hide.

Why didn't I get caught?

Because ***Baric gave me legal invisibility***.

Until ***someone ran the right alignment tool***.

And saw ***our names in the genome***.

The Virus Had to Be Natural—So the Vaccine Could Be Righteous

Here's the trick.

You can't run ***global human trials***
on a virus ***you engineered***.

Not publicly.

Not ethically.

Not ***without the world asking questions we weren't prepared to answer***.

So we needed something more than a vaccine.

We needed ***a myth***.

And no-see-um gave us one.

Because if the virus ***looked natural***—
then the vaccine was ***a gift***.

A miracle.
A product of ingenuity.
The solution to ***an act of God***.

Not ***an act of us***.

You think Pfizer wanted to ask where the spike protein came from?

You think Moderna wanted to put "recombinant ferret-adapted chimera" in their SEC filings?

Come on.

They wanted ***clean deliverables***.

Clean funding.
Clean ethics board approvals.
Clean indemnity.

And we gave it to them.

With ***a codon-optimized lie***.

The moment we labeled SARS-CoV-2 “natural,”
we opened the door to ***everything else***.

- Emergency Use Authorization
- Accelerated human trials
- Pre-purchased doses
- Platform testing
- mRNA normalization
- Liability shields

You can’t grant EUA for a ***manmade virus from a classified research pipeline***.

But for ***a zoonotic spillover***?

Go for it.

No one gets sued.

No one gets questioned.

No one goes to jail.

That's what no-see-um protected:

Not just ***the method***—

But ***the response***.

The ***entire apparatus*** rested on the premise that:

"This virus caught us by surprise."

So we needed ***speed***.

And ***trust***.

And ***cooperation***.

And ***no autopsies***.

If it had looked synthetic?

Everything stops.

The whole machine freezes.

Because suddenly:

- Every trial is suspect
- Every subject is a potential victim
- Every company is complicit
- Every agency is implicated

You don't get a global platform test.

You get ***Geneva***.

So no-see-um?

It wasn't just molecular sleight of hand.

It was ***narrative infrastructure***:

The only thing standing between:

- ***A miracle vaccine rollout***

and

- ***A tribunal.***

By the way, I didn't fake the trials.

I faked ***the origin***.

So the trials could go forward without anyone asking:

"What exactly are we curing?"

The Technique Was the Real Pandemic

You want to know what spread faster than SARS-CoV-2?

Baric's method.

The paper came out.
The ligation maps.
The protocols.
The ***how-to guide on hiding a synthetic virus*** in plain sight.

And suddenly?

Everyone had a ***no-see-um kit***.

Wuhan?
Obviously.

They were ***co-listed*** on the original gain-of-function collaborations.

They didn't need to reverse-engineer the method.

They ***helped build it***.

But then it spread.

Utrecht.
Duke-NUS in Singapore.
Hong Kong University.
INSERM in France.
Charité in Berlin.
Even a couple labs in Ukraine.

We trained them.
We published with them.
We ***shared the method like it was a vaccine***.

And guess what?

It ***was***.

A ***vaccine for accountability***.

You use no-see-um?

You get ***invisibility by design***.

Not just from regulators.

From ***your peers***.

Because if the data looks clean?

Nobody asks what you left out.

That's what made it dangerous.

Not the viruses it built.

But ***the culture it created***.

A generation of virologists raised on the idea that ***proof of natural origin was optional—so long as the genome didn't snitch***.

And here's where it gets ugly.

Once everyone was using the same method?

You couldn't trace ***anything***.

Too many hands.
Too many labs.
Too many overlaps.

Even I ***couldn't follow it after a point***.

You ask me where SARS-CoV-2 was built?

I could give you five cities.

Three labs.

And ***one method*** that made them all indistinguishable.

We didn't globalize the virus.

We globalized ***the cover story***.

And it worked.

Until someone looked too closely.

I didn't create a virus.

I ***licensed a technique***.

And once it was out?

Every lab became ***a potential patient zero***.

Which means ***none of them were***.

That's the trick.

That's the beauty.

That's ***no-see-um***.

When Everyone's Guilty, You Pick the Enemy

Once no-see-um went global?

Nobody could say where anything came from.

So we made a choice:

We picked **Wuhan**.

Not because it was innocent.
Not because it was guilty.
Because it was ***convenient***.

They had:

- The samples
- The funding trail
- The bat caves
- The Chinese firewall
- The optics of secrecy
- The right amount of blame-worthiness
- And ***none of the power to fight back***.

Perfect scapegoat.

Not too clean.
Not too strong.
Not too clear.

Just ***gray enough to absorb it***.

You think we couldn't have pointed the finger at ***UNC***?

Where Baric ran the templates?

Where we ran ***live animal passage experiments*** before DEFUSE was even written?

Sure we could've.

But that's ***home soil***.

Too messy.

We could've pointed at **Charité in Germany**.

Where early spike modeling was happening.
Where Baric's collaborators tested ***immune escape variants***.

But they're ***EU***.
They were ***good soldiers***.

Too useful.

Wuhan?

That's ***China***.

Built-in plausibility.

Built-in mistrust.

Built-in censorship.

We didn't even have to say much.

We just had to let ***others*** say it.

And we ***didn't contradict them***.

That's all it took.

Once the world started chanting ***"lab leak,"***
we said:

"Maybe. Probably not. Let's investigate later."

Which meant:

"Yes. But let's make sure ***no one looks at the rest of us***."

The truth?

Wuhan was part of it.
But so were we.
So were ***they***.

It wasn't ***a conspiracy***.

It was ***a professional courtesy***.

Everyone used the method.
So ***nobody wanted the method on trial***.

Just ***the lab***.

And by keeping the focus there?

We ***preserved the system***.

The funding.
The journals.
The partnerships.
The ***next round of research***.

Wuhan became ***the firewall***.

So the real fire wouldn't touch ***the rest of us***.

We Didn't Just Escape—We Accelerated

Wuhan didn't end the conversation.

It ***supercharged it***.

Because once the world settled on a villain?

We got to ***write the rest of the story***.

The virus was real.
The danger was real.
The origin? ***Ambiguous***.

Perfect.

Because ambiguity gives you ***leverage***.

And leverage?

Gives you ***time***.

We used that time well.

- **Emergency declarations**
- **Funding boosts**
- **Censorship partnerships**
- **Fast-tracked approvals**
- **New mRNA platforms**
- **Global digital ID infrastructure**

That didn't come from a pandemic.

It came from ***DEFUSE***.

And from ***the void*** we left behind it.

Let me be blunt:

Without DEFUSE?

There is no:

- Warp Speed
- Boosters
- Immunity passports
- Social media “trusted flagger” systems
- Spike-protein-as-a-platform business model
- ***Next generation vaccine pipeline***

And no ***pre-cleared runway for the next outbreak***.

We didn’t just cover our tracks.

We ***laid new ones***.

While everyone was still arguing about bats in wet markets, we were ***writing contracts***.

Pfizer.
Moderna.
CEPI.
GAVI.
WHO.

The map was already drawn.

We just had to ***burn the origin site*** long enough for no one to look behind us.

And it worked.

You know how I know?

Because ***DEFUSE 2.0 is already drafted***.

New viruses.
New partners.
Same excuses.

All under **"global biosecurity."**

We didn't end gain-of-function.

We ***globalized*** it.

And made it ***indispensable***.

That's the legacy of DEFUSE.

Not a leak.

A ***framework***.

That scaled globally.

Because ***the method was portable***.
And the panic?
Reusable.

I ***built the future*** using ***the fire we lit***.

And when the smoke cleared?

I wasn't hiding.

I was ***at the podium***.

Smiling.

While the next proposal slid across a desk
with ***better fonts and a bigger budget***.

I Stayed So They Didn't Have To

You want to know why I didn't resign?

Why I stood behind the podium
week after week,
variant after variant,
while everyone else disappeared into consulting gigs and substack exile?

Because ***someone had to stay visible***.

And they promised ***I'd be protected***.

Not publicly.
Not in writing.

Just understood.

Hold the line.

So the others could reset.

Take the blame.

So the system could move forward.

Be ***the face***.
So ***the machine*** wouldn't show its real one.

And I did it.

Not for the science.
Not even for the money.

For ***continuity***.

Because ***if I disappeared***,
too many eyes would've turned ***the wrong direction***.

Back to UNC.
Back to EcoHealth.
Back to ***DEFUSE***.

So I played the role.

Doctor.
Advisor.
Martyr.
Villain.
Saint.
Punching bag.

Whatever was needed that week.

And I took it.

Every interview.
Every leak.
Every Senate grilling.
Every FOIA dump.
Every podcast ambush.
Every death threat.
Every meme.

I even took ***the autopen***.

Yeah.

Let's talk about that.

You know what they promised me?

"We'll make sure it's handled."

And it was.

But not like I thought.

Not like ***Hunter***.

He got the full treatment.

Real signature.
Real document.
Real ***quiet***.

Me?

They printed mine out.
Stamped it with ***a robot pen***.

"Don't take it personal, Tony."

But I did.

Because after everything I shielded,
after everyone I covered for—

They sent me home with a machine-written fuck you.

I didn't ask for a monument.

I just thought ***Biden would sign his name*** when they cut me loose.

Instead?

Click. Buzz. Done.

That's all I got.

From a system I kept standing
while everyone else ***walked away clean***.

Until now.

He should have signed my name in ink.

CHAPTER 4

They Didn't Follow the Science— They Followed Me

La Science, C'est Moi.

From the outside, it looked like a consensus.
Public health officials.
University deans.
Tech platforms.
Global leaders.

Everyone marching to the same beat.

"Trust the science."
"Follow the data."
"Do what Fauci says."

And for a while, I believed it too.
I thought they were following **the science**.

But they weren't.

They were following **me**.

You want to know what science actually looks like?

It's messy.
It contradicts itself.
It gets things wrong and corrects them years later—*quietly*, in footnotes.

But that doesn't sell.
That doesn't work on CNN.
That doesn't get you 70% compliance in a population that can't agree on how to toast bread.

So instead of science, we created a **symbol**.

And that symbol was me.

They made me the North Star.
The last word.
The oracle.

And I went along with it.

I sat for interviews.
I threw out crisp numbers.
I projected certainty on things I only half-believed that morning.
Not because I was lying—
but because I knew the **public didn't want doubt**.

They wanted guidance.
They wanted clarity.
They wanted to *believe* that someone had this under control.

So I gave it to them.

But here's the problem:

Once you become the face of The Science™,
you can't ever say **you were wrong**.

Because if I'm wrong, then maybe the mandates were wrong.
Maybe the school closures were wrong.
Maybe the vaccines weren't tested the way we said.
Maybe the origin wasn't natural.
Maybe the whole thing wasn't what we claimed.

And if that dam breaks—
everything floods.

So instead of reassessing, we **doubled down**.

- We told people who got sick after three shots that they were still "better off."

- We told parents their toddlers needed masks but said nothing about playgrounds.
- We banned dissent, not because it was false, but because it was *inconvenient*.

And we told ourselves we were saving lives.

They say "science isn't a person."
True.

But in 2020, it became one.
It became **me**.

That's not arrogance.
That's what we designed.

The system needed a singular voice—
someone to project stability into the chaos.

And I fit the mold.

The irony?

I never wanted that kind of power.
But once I had it…
I didn't exactly hand it back either.

I did it because everyone else needed me to.

And once the myth was built—
that **I was the science**—
it didn't matter what the actual data said.

It only mattered what *I* said it said.

And if you still think that's science?

I've got a mask mandate to sell you.

CHAPTER 5

The Mask Slipped, Didn't It?

Let's talk about masks.

Not the science. Not the mandates.
Not the fact that every CVS in America became a surgical supply depot overnight.
Let's talk about the theater.

Because that's what it became.
And honestly? I helped write the script.

Back in March 2020, I said masks don't work.
You've probably seen the clip. Grainy, fast-talking, me waving my hands: "There's no reason to be walking around with a mask."
It's true. I said that.

And then, weeks later, I said the opposite.
Not because the virus changed.
Not because the studies changed.
But because **the narrative needed to**.

The dirty secret about masks is this:
It was never just about blocking a virus.
It was about sending a signal.

If I tell the country to wear masks, I'm telling them: *this is serious.*
If I tell them not to, I'm saying: *this will pass.*

In early 2020, we needed calm.
We needed compliance for things that actually mattered—like stockpiling PPE for hospitals, not hoarding it for brunch.

So I lied.
Yes. That's what it was.
A tactical misdirection.
Not "the science evolved."
Not "we learned more."
Just a decision: **they're not ready**.

Later, I said I was "trying to preserve supply."
Which is true. But it wasn't the whole truth.

By April, everything flipped.
Masks became sacred.
Not because they suddenly worked better—but because **they were a unifying ritual**.

We turned them into **totems**.

Wear the mask, and you're on the side of science.
Don't, and you're a COVID-denying lunatic who probably drinks horse paste and watches Tucker on a loop.

The nuance was gone.
Cloth masks? Didn't matter.
Neck gaiters, surgical blue, homemade flannel with dog bones on them? Irrelevant.

Effectiveness was secondary.
Allegiance was the point.

Did they help? Sometimes. A little. Maybe.

If you had a tight-fitting N95, sealed properly, with facial hair trimmed and no gaps, and you wore it indoors consistently, sure.
That helps. Unless you touch your face. Hah.
But that's not what most people were doing.
They were reusing cotton cloths they found in a glove box.

We knew that.
We just couldn't *say* that.

Because if we admitted the marginal utility, we'd lose the ritual.

And rituals are **powerful**.

Here's what I learned from masks:
A symbol is stronger than a fact.

I could show people airflow diagrams, explain droplet physics, cite aerosol filtration studies. But the moment someone sees a nurse in a mask or a grocery clerk behind a plexiglass shield, they don't want science.
They want certainty.
They want to feel like they're *doing something*.

Masks gave people that.

For some, they were talismans.
For others, they were muzzles.
For politicians? They were polling tools.

For me?
They were… a lever.
Push it one way, you get fear. Push it another, you get discipline.

Push it hard enough, you get obedience.

Was it manipulative? Yes.
Was it necessary? You tell me.

When you're managing a nation of 330 million during a fog-of-war biological event, you don't always get to be honest.

Sometimes, you just need them to *comply*.

That's what masks were for.

And then, when we said *two* masks were better?
That wasn't science either.
That was just panic with a fabric budget.

Now I see people wearing them alone in cars.
I see kids masked on playgrounds, three feet apart, in the sun.
I see joggers gasping through wet cloth in empty parks.

That's not protection.
That's the **residue of propaganda**.

Mine.
Ours.
Everyone's.

I did it because I thought it would help. And then I did it because I couldn't stop.
Because once you pull the mask over their face…
it's very, very hard to take it off.

And even harder to admit why you put it there.

CHAPTER 6

Six Feet Apart Was Made Up

Let's settle this once and for all:

Six feet apart wasn't science.
It was **guesswork**.

Polished, packaged, and sold as certainty because someone needed a number—and **six** felt authoritative.

Not five. Too soft.
Not seven. Too weird.
Six. Solid. Presidential.

We needed something that could fit on a laminated floor sticker.

The idea came from **decades-old studies** on respiratory droplet spread.
Back when the only viruses we modeled were measles, TB, and what your grandmother called "the grippe."

Most of the data?
Pre-1960s.
No controlled trials.
No high-speed aerosol imaging.
Just: sneezes go this far, probably.

Did we revise it for COVID?

Of course not.

We had **days** to turn centuries of microbiology into public policy. So we took the old number, stripped the context, doubled the font size, and sent it to every school, airport, and Waffle House in America.

The truth?

COVID isn't a droplet virus. Not really.

It's **aerosolized**.

That means the virus floats in the air like cigarette smoke.
Six feet doesn't matter when the particles hang around for **hours** in a poorly ventilated room.

But saying that would've required us to admit two uncomfortable things:

1. Most indoor spaces were **unsafe**, no matter the sticker on the floor.

2. The only real mitigation was **ventilation and filtration**, which is expensive, slow, and doesn't look good in a press conference.

So we stuck with six feet.

Because it was simple.
Because it was cheap.
Because it looked like action.

When schools reopened, we told kids to space out their desks by six feet.
When that made classrooms unusable, we said **three feet was okay**—overnight, with no new data.

And just like that, the science "evolved."

You want to know what *actually* evolved? The political calculus.

We told couples they had to sit six feet apart in restaurants but could go home and sleep together.
We told churches to block off pews but let people pack into subways.
We let airlines fill every seat in coach, because the **air filtration systems** on planes are "superior."

Sure. And the peanuts are sterile too, I'm sure.

The problem wasn't the rule.
It was the **illusion of precision**.

People thought six feet was a force field.
They'd lean into conversations at five feet eleven like they were safe, but explode in panic if someone stepped inside that imaginary radius.

We built a public health strategy on **imaginary geometry**.

We were playing *The Floor Is Lava*—except the floor was air, and lava was everywhere.

I made up six feet because people needed *something*.
A number. A rule. A ritual.

And maybe that's the worst part.

Because once you start inventing numbers to calm the mob, it gets harder and harder to stop.

CHAPTER 7

Omertà

Lab Coat Mafia: Why Scientists Don't Snitch

You want to know why nobody ever blew the whistle?

Nobody leaked the raw sequences.
Nobody forwarded the DEFUSE proposal to a real journalist.
Nobody stood up in front of a Senate hearing and said, "*We made it. We screwed up.*"

I'll tell you why:

Because science—at this level—isn't peer review.
It's **omertà**.

And the guys in the white coats?
They don't snitch.

In public, science sells itself as open. Transparent. Self-correcting.

But at the top?
It's a **closed guild**.

You publish each other.
You review each other's grants.
You sit on the same panels, attend the same retreats, co-author each other's *Nature* pieces.

You call it collegiality.
I call it **non-denominational Freemasonry with pipettes**.

You know how many people it took to build SARS-CoV-2—if it was built?

Dozens.
Maybe more.
You've got:

- The genome modelers
- The sequence jockeys
- The postdocs pipetting furin sites into replicons
- The field teams trapping bats

- The spillover "modelers" whose job is to simulate what you're already doing in real life

And not **one** of them talked?

Correct.
Because they know the rules.

Rule #1: **You don't jeopardize the grant**.
Rule #2: **You don't burn a co-author**.
Rule #3: **You don't give the House Energy & Commerce Committee anything they can understand**.

Let's be honest:
We all knew what EcoHealth was doing.
We all read Baric's papers.
We all saw Fouchier's ferret experiments.

We just **didn't call it what it was**.

We called it "predictive virology."
We called it "pandemic preparedness."
We called it "constructive ambiguity."

In any other context, it would've been called weapons prototyping. But we were wearing lab coats instead of fatigues, so it got a pass.

Why didn't someone stop it?

Because they were **in on it**.
Or they were funded by it.
Or they were *next in line* for a spot on the next blue-ribbon panel, with a check waiting just past the revolving door.

You blow the whistle on this stuff and you don't just lose your job.
You lose your publishing career.
Your tenure track.
Your invitations to Davos.

You get labeled a crank, a "conspiracy theorist," or worse: a bad collaborator.

Remember when *The Lancet* letter came out in early 2020?
The one that slammed the "lab leak theory" as "dangerous misinformation"?

Every signatory had a conflict.
Every one of them stood to lose funding, access, prestige.

But they signed anyway.

Because the **Lab Coat Mafia sticks together**.

We don't rat.
We cite.

And when the backlash started—when people began asking real questions—what did we do?

We didn't answer.

We **coordinated**.

Zoom calls. Pre-drafted statements. Peer-reviewed firewall articles written faster than most of us could finish a coffee.

We circled the wagons, not because we had proof...
but because **proof wasn't the point anymore**.

Control was.

And if you think I'm the only one who should've talked?

Well then, you've never met a virologist with a DoD contract and a family mortgage in Bethesda. They all knew.

And they all shut up.

Because that’s the rule.

CHAPTER 8

Run, Death Is Near

Remdesivir.
Sounds futuristic, right?

It killed 53% of Ebola patients.
So we knew it was powerful.

Didn't work in Africa.
Too lethal.
Too unethical.
The trial got shut down.

But COVID wasn't Ebola.
Different branding.
Different budget.
Different incentives.

I said it would work.
I said it early.
I said it loud.

It didn't stop COVID.
But it stopped kidneys.
Then it stopped livers.
Then it stopped hearts.

Ventilator + Remdesivir =
Pulmonary edema.
Patients drown in their own lungs.

That's not COVID.
That's protocol.

And we paid for it.
20% hospital bonus if they used it.
Not for saving lives.
Just for administering it.
Death by spreadsheet.

The WHO eventually said:
"Do not use Remdesivir."
We said:
"Use it more. On babies."

Infants. Neonates.
FDA approved.
Fast-tracked in under 3 years.
Normally takes ten.

Why wait?
No liability. No resistance.
Just trust the science.

It's still in hospitals today.
Still on protocols.
Still has that kill rate problem.
But now it's got a marketing team.

"Veklury."
Sounds like a skincare brand.
Kills like a chemical weapon.

The Only Approved Drug Money Could Buy

Remdesivir wasn't just a treatment.
It was **an asset**.

The NIH had a stake.
A real, financial stake.
Not just funding.
Royalties.
Cut of the pie.

That's what made it different.
That's why it was **allowed**.

Hydroxychloroquine?
No stake.
Ivermectin?
Generic. Cheap.
No upside.

Remdesivir?
Patented.
Expensive.
Proprietary.
Ours.

And that *Ebola trial*?
Sure, it killed more people than it cured.
But we had **"data."**
And I had a narrative.

SCENE: Oval Office Press Conference — April 2020

Me. Standing there.
White House backdrop.
Mask off, spine straight, voice calibrated.

I said:

"Remdesivir has a clear-cut, significant, positive effect."

Said it with conviction.
Didn't mention the 53% mortality in Ebola.
Didn't mention **the kidney failure**.
Didn't mention the **conflict of interest** with the clinical trial investigators—
Same guys who *slammed* HCQ and IVM?
Also running the Remdesivir trials.
Go figure.

I sold it.
Like it was the moon landing.

Cut to Trump.
Next to me.
Looking like a guy who just realized he's in the back seat of his own car.

His face said:
"Wait… did we just bet the whole pandemic on a drug that melts kidneys?"
But his mouth said:

"That's a big statement."
"That's a very positive event."

He trusted me.
For ten minutes.
That's all I needed.

Remdesivir was never about treatment.
It was about control.
It was **approved. Promoted. Incentivized.**
Because it was ours.

The only antiviral we could monetize.
Not the best. Just the best-connected.

And if a few kidneys got shredded along the way?
We called that **secondary endpoints**.

Next slide.

From AZT to Remdesivir to Paxlovid: A Tradition of Toxic Excellence

I have a *type*.
Toxic. Expensive. Immune-destroying.
And fully indemnified.

First, there was **AZT**.
The original star.
Approved in *record time* for HIV.
Destroyed bone marrow.
Killed faster than the virus.

But it made headlines.
And billions.

It wasn't about helping.
It was about **owning the protocol**.
And shutting down anything cheap.
Anything that worked too well.

Same script. New pathogen.

Fast forward:
Remdesivir.
Another nucleoside analog. Another failed antiviral.
Another **deadly repurpose** with a new PR team.

Didn't cure Ebola.
Didn't cure COVID.
But it did one thing perfectly:
Locked in the hospital system.

Now we've got Paxlovid.
Pfizer's golden boy.
$530 per treatment.
And guess what's in it?
A *protease inhibitor.*
Just like AZT's cousins.
Same class of drugs.
Same playbook.

And the best part?
It **rebound infects**.
Virus comes back stronger.
So we tell people:
"Just take another course."

That's not failure.
That's **subscription-based medicine**.

Judy Mikovits tried to warn people.
She talked about **immune collapse, viral reactivation, latent infections**.
Said AZT wrecked the immune system.
Said Remdesivir was the **same molecular scam**.
Said Paxlovid would **retrigger** chronic disease in people with viral baggage.

I said she was crazy.
And then I made sure she stayed unemployed.

Because here's the thing—
None of this is new.
It's a franchise.
AZT. Remdesivir. Paxlovid.

You don't retire a poison that still pays.
You rebrand it.
You fast-track it.
You give it to kids.

Then you call it **progress**.

Next patient.

Full Circle

I've been trying to make this work since **1987**.
AZT.
The first time I bet the house on a toxic antiviral.

Back then, they said I rushed it.
Said it was dangerous.
Said I killed people.

Same story. Different virus.
But I don't quit.

One of my greatest strengths?
I'm never wrong—
if I keep going long enough.

Because success isn't about outcomes.
It's about *survival.*
Staying in the room longer than your critics.
Let the bodies fall where they may.
I'm still standing.

So now, with Remdesivir still in hospitals…
With Paxlovid in every pharmacy…
With kids getting fast-tracked poison wrapped in a $500 price tag…

That's not failure.
That's not tragedy.
That's vindication.

It means I was right.
It always meant I was right.

Eventually.

Next crisis.

Monoclones and Money Clones

Monoclonal antibodies.
They worked.
That was the problem.

Neutralized the spike.
Reduced hospitalizations.
People got better. Too fast.

Couldn't have that.
Not while we were pushing *Remdesivir*.
Not while *Paxlovid* was still in the oven.

So we came up with a phrase:
"No longer authorized."

Not because they didn't work.
But because they didn't work *against new variants.*
(That we never clinically tested them on.)

Science.

Florida kept using them.
DeSantis had those mobile units.
People lined up—
and walked away healthy.

Bad optics.
We needed *deaths* to justify the *emergency.*
So we pulled the plug.

"Sorry, no more EUAs."
Not because they failed.
But because **they weren't ours**.

You want to know how fast we moved?
We shut down Regeneron and Lilly's antibodies in **under 24 hours**. **Millions of doses. Canceled. Trashed.**

Because when it came time to choose between:
A. Saving lives, or
B. Preserving the narrative,

We chose B. Every time.

We said:

"They don't neutralize Omicron."
Even though we had no human data.
No trial.
No dose-response.

Just a model.
A pseudovirus.
A lab guess.

And we ran with it.
Shut it all down.

Why?
Because monoclonals were a **threat to the protocol**.
Too effective.
Too fast.
Too unprofitable.

We needed hospital beds full.
We needed prescriptions.
We didn't need cures.

That's the game.
Not about helping.
About **managing**.

Monoclonals helped people escape the maze.
So we bricked the exits.

Monoclonals were safe.
Effective.
Fast.

And unpatentable.
And politically inconvenient.
So we killed them.

We needed sick people.
We needed protocols.
We didn't need cures.

What no one tells you?
Monoclonals even helped **Long COVID**.
Yeah.

European studies showed improvement.
Reduced inflammation.
Cleared persistent spike debris.
Patients stabilized.

Approved in the EU.
Not here.

We couldn't risk that.
Couldn't admit there *was* a lingering spike protein problem—
Because that would raise the obvious question:

Where's all that spike coming from?
Hmmm.

Let's just say:
Long COVID does seem to show up more in the **vaccinated**.

Coincidence.
Let's not get into it.

I'd love to talk about it.
Really.

But I'm gonna need a **second pardon** for that conversation.

CHAPTER 9
The Revolving Door and the Golden Needle

Let's stop pretending there's a wall between public health and Big Pharma. There's a **revolving door**—so well-oiled you don't even hear it spin.

You spend twenty years approving grants, designing clinical trials, and shaping public messaging, and then—when it's time to "retire"—you walk straight into a board seat, a consulting gig, or a $200k keynote at a biotech summit.

They call it a "transition."
I call it a **golden needle**:
Your reward for keeping the machine humming.

I know how this looks.

A guy like me—government job, modest salary, big public trust. You'd think I was immune to influence.

But here's the real inoculation:
career capital.

Every piece of funding I approved...
every trial I greenlit...
every researcher I vouched for...

All of that **accumulates value**—not just in lives, but in *equity.*

Scientific equity.
Policy equity.
Actual equity, if you play your cards right.

You want to know how this works?

Here's the three-step process:

1. **Public Money Builds the Tool**.
    - NIAID funds the platform (mRNA, protein subunit, viral vector).
    - NIH researchers develop the early-stage tech.
    - Taxpayer dollars bankroll basic science with "no commercial bias."
2. **Private Companies Weaponize the Tool**.
    - Moderna, BioNTech, Pfizer, Sanofi license the tech.
    - They get fast-tracked approval with friendly FDA contacts.
    - We let them patent improvements built off public research.
3. **The Architects Cash Out**.
    - Founders retire.
    - Advisors get stock options.
    - Former agency heads consult "off the record."

- NIH scientists collect royalties—quietly—on the very patents they helped approve.
- The regulators become the stakeholders.
- And nobody recuses.

Wash. Rinse. Booster.

During the pandemic, Moderna minted billionaires.
Pfizer rewrote history books.
BioNTech turned a startup into a geopolitical power broker.

And what did we say?

"We're saving lives."

Well, maybe.
But we were also **pricing third-world nations out of the market**,
locking countries into subscription models,
and building a global dependency on private vaccine IP.

You think we were trying to "end the pandemic"? No.
We were **monetizing it**.

Every CEO has my number.
Every pharma roundtable wants a piece of the action.

And now that I'm out?

Now that I've testified, spun, survived, and held the line?

Let's just say the **consulting calendar is filling up fast**.

You want to know why no one blew the whistle on mRNA trial irregularities?
On the fact that **Pfizer's trials never even measured transmission**?
On the endless redefinition of "efficacy"?

Because everyone was **positioning for the pivot**.

You keep your head down, you get your post.
You don't ask about myocarditis rates or adverse event curves—you ask about the equity package.

And when the dust settles?

You say it was all "in the interest of public health."

Because who's going to argue with that?

I didn't just help make the narrative.
I helped make the **market**.

And when the pandemic ends, the story does too.

But the stock options?
Those keep vesting.

CHAPTER 10

We Had a Narrative, and It Was Too Beautiful to Break

By now, maybe you understand:
This was never just a public health crisis.
It was a **narrative event**.

A story so perfectly structured, so emotionally satisfying, so **morally engineered**, that it didn't matter if it was true.

What mattered was that it **worked**.

The virus had a villain: nature.
A savior: the scientists.
A simple fix: masks, distance, lockdown.
A heroic climax: a vaccine, faster than ever before.
And a final moral: trust the experts, even when they contradict themselves.

Hollywood couldn't have done it better.

And when people started asking questions—about origins, gain-of-function, myocarditis, PCR cycle thresholds—we didn't just dismiss them.

We **silenced** them.

Because if they were right, even a little...
then the whole story started to collapse.

And the one thing worse than a broken system?

A broken myth.

So we kept going.

We leaned on platforms to de-rank dissent.
We rewrote definitions—of "vaccine," of "immunity," of "case."
We promoted spokespeople who smiled on camera and nodded like priests.

Every contradiction—"two weeks to flatten the curve," "you won't get infected if you're vaccinated," "masks don't work / masks save lives"—wasn't a bug.
It was a **plot twist**.

And the public?
They *wanted* the plot twist.
They wanted the experts to win.

Even when the data said otherwise.

Especially then.

We didn't lie for profit.
We lied for **stability**.
For order.
For control.

And then—when the cracks started to show—we told ourselves it was **too late** to go back.

What were we going to do?
Tell the world the origin was probably a lab?
That the vaccine trials were never designed to
measure transmission?
That school closures didn't stop spread but did spike suicide rates and developmental delays?

No.

Because we had a story.

And it was too **big to fail**.

CHAPTER 11

The PREDICT Pipeline

How We Fed the Dragon and Called It Prevention

You want to know how it got to Wuhan?

Here's your answer.

Not through espionage.
Not through wet markets.
Not even through EcoHealth—at least, not directly.

It got there through a **State Department–funded program** called **PREDICT**.

Run by USAID.
Administered by UC Davis.
Promoted as wildlife surveillance.
In practice? A **pathogen supply chain**.

Between 2009 and 2019, we funneled **over 11,000 virus samples**—collected from bats, rodents, primates, livestock—into **foreign labs**, including the **Wuhan Institute of Virology**.

That's not a conspiracy theory.

That's the paperwork.

The PREDICT field teams collected samples in **Yunnan Province**, an area already known for harboring bat coronaviruses *very close to SARS-CoV-2.*

And instead of storing them in U.S. labs?
We sent them **to Wuhan**.

There was no backup archive.
No formal storage agreement.
No inspection protocol.
Just boxes of frozen pathogens flown into a lab with **known military ties** and **a leaky safety record**.

Why?

Because we were told it was about **collaboration**.
"Global health diplomacy."
"Capacity building."

But what it really was?

Outsourcing risk.

Wuhan had fewer rules.
Fewer lawyers.
Fewer watchdogs.

And we had a diplomatic shield:
"This is just research."

Let's talk about who was involved:

- **USAID** wrote the checks.
- **UC Davis** ran point.
- **EcoHealth Alliance** acted as the middleman, coordinating sampling and sequence analysis.
- **Metabiota**, a biotech firm tied to U.S. defense and intel contracts, ran field logistics.
- **WIV** received, stored, and analyzed the samples—often under opaque, military-influenced conditions.

We called it a virome survey.

But in effect?
It was a **virus export program**—with **no downstream control**.

I've read the reports.

The language is always the same:

"Samples collected in Yunnan were sent to, tested, and stored in Wuhan."

"No duplicate sample archive exists in U.S. facilities."

"No formal agreement governs biosafety standards or data retention."

We gave them the raw material.

And then we acted shocked when something **novel** came back.

You want the part no one wants to say?

We didn't even know what we gave them.

These weren't just labeled vials.

They were **highly recombinant-capable pathogens**, many of them undocumented, uncharacterized, and shipped overseas **without a chain of custody**.

And we called that "science."

We didn't just fund Wuhan.

We stocked it.

Why?

Because it was cleaner than doing it at home.
Because the Pentagon didn't want a domestic trail.
Because the intel community saw virology as **soft surveillance**—a way to access regions they couldn't touch with satellites and drones.

PREDICT was pitched as global health.
But it functioned like **bio-distribution with diplomatic cover**.

And the worst part?

It worked.

Until one of the samples, or one of the experiments, or one of the accidents turned into something that *couldn't be walked back.*

The things I did, I did by signing off on the system.
Not the leak.
The **pipeline**.

And once it was running?

Nobody—especially not me—was going to shut it off.

Let's talk about the logistics arm.

The people who actually handled the field teams, the databases, the coordination between jungle sampling sites and military-linked labs.

That was **Metabiota**.

If EcoHealth was the virology middleman, Metabiota was the **bagman with a clipboard**.

Officially, they were "disease modelers" and "outbreak risk analysts."
In practice, they were the ones **moving the samples**—quietly, globally, and with near-zero visibility.

And here's where it gets even more convenient:

Metabiota was backed by Rosemont Seneca.
As in, **Hunter Biden's venture capital firm**.

The same Rosemont Seneca that was plugged into the U.S. intelligence ecosystem, Ukrainian energy deals, and global development funds.

A biotech startup with a foot in PREDICT's viral pipeline—and a financial umbilical cord to the son of a sitting Vice President?

That's not just funding.

That's **cover**.

Try raising alarms about a private contractor's overseas virus collection program when it's **co-owned by the guy one heartbeat away from the Oval Office**.

You won't get far.

Not in 2014.
Not in 2016.
Not when everyone's betting on global health as the next frontier of "resilience investment."

Was Hunter sequencing bat viruses?

No.

But his name on the cap table meant **no one was going to shut this thing down**.
Not USAID.
Not DTRA.
Not NIH.
Not the White House, that's for damn sure.

So Metabiota kept running samples.
From caves in Yunnan
to freezers in Wuhan
to *god knows where* after that.

And nobody asked questions—
because they already knew **whose project it was**.

I didn't just build the pipeline.
I watched people use it to move **the most dangerous material on earth**, and smiled—
because they said it was for peace.

And because the **right names were on the letterhead**.

CHAPTER 12

They Always Knew

You Don't Hide a Machine Like This—You Just Don't Look at It Directly

You think this was a secret?

It wasn't.

The people who needed to know—**knew**.
And the people who didn't?
Made damn sure not to ask.

Because once you *know*, you can't un-know.
And if you know and **do nothing**—you're now part of it.

So everyone played dumb.

Strategically.

The State Department?
They got cables in 2018 warning that the Wuhan Institute of Virology had military ties and subpar biosafety protocols.

The Pentagon?
They were funding EcoHealth through DTRA and backing Metabiota through USAID. DoD knew exactly what was being built—and **where the samples were going**.

NIH?
We reviewed the proposals.
We saw the overlap between "pandemic prevention" and **offensive virology capabilities**.
We didn't reject them.

Because if we did, we'd have to explain **why we were funding them in the first place**.

And the intelligence community?

They weren't in the dark.
They were in the loop.

PREDICT wasn't just a health program.
It was a **strategic access platform**.
We used disease surveillance to map wildlife viromes **and local infrastructure** in regions we couldn't otherwise touch.

The virus was the pretext.

The movement of people, money, and materials—that was the real value.

And if you think CIA didn't know that EcoHealth was funneling samples to a military-adjacent lab in Wuhan?

Then you don't know how intel works.

Even the *White House* knew.

Not the interns.
Not the speechwriters.

The real operators.
The National Security Council types.
The people who sit in on meetings and **never show up in photos**.

They saw the briefings.
They read the biosafety assessments.
They knew what PREDICT really was.

And they didn't stop it.

Because **it was working**.

Until it wasn't.

No one had to lie.

All they had to do was look away.
Delay the emails.
Let the grants renew.
Use the right language.

Words like "spillover," "resilience," "preparedness."
Words that sound like strategy but function like fog.

And in that fog,
we built the most dangerous virology pipeline in history.

Out in the open.

And I didn't do it alone.
I did it with a network of very smart people who knew how to protect the system—

By pretending they didn't know exactly what it was.

CHAPTER 13

Science Is a Scam

Science Is the Only Religion Where the Priests Don't Know They're Priests

Look.

I'm going to tell you something no one in a white coat is ever supposed to say.

Science is a scam.

Not all of it.

Just… the part people listen to.

You think "peer-reviewed" means verified? No.

It means a guy you met at a conference in Belgium owes you a favor.
It means the paper didn't contradict too many grant assumptions.
It means the results matched the *narrative*.
It means **the editors weren't scared of the fallout**.

You publish what you're allowed to.
And when you can't publish it?

It never happened.

We delete the bad studies.

We hide the null results.

We ghostwrite pharma-funded conclusions.

We add three co-authors to keep the citations flowing and the university chair happy.

You think that paper in *Nature* is the product of months of clean, replicable inquiry?

It's a **press release** in a lab coat.

Why do we give Nobel Prizes to mRNA inventors
then ban doctors for mentioning natural immunity?

Because **you're not supposed to see it**.

You're only supposed to believe it.

Science doesn't prove anything.

That's the trick.

It just keeps pushing the burden of proof further away from you.

You see something with your own eyes?

Doesn't matter.

Unless you have a cohort study, 36-month follow-up, and a p-value under 0.05—
you're the crank.

Even if I'm lying.

Especially if I'm lying.

We set the standard so high,
you can never accuse us of anything.

Ever.

You say, "This spike protein seems engineered."

We say: "Prove it."

You say, "This policy's killing kids."

We say: "Where's your RCT?"

You say, "This lab leaked a virus."

We say: "Not conclusive. Also, you're a conspiracy theorist."

You see how it works?

We don't have to win.
We just make **certainty impossible** for everyone but us.

The courtroom says, "beyond reasonable doubt."

Science says, "beyond reproducible probability, adjusted for confounders, unless retracted in a paywalled journal two years later."

Good luck with that.

You want truth?

You're in the wrong building.

Science doesn't give you truth.

It gives you **authority**.

And the more uncertain we are,
the more certain we have to sound.

Look.

I already told you: **science is a scam**.

But it's not a solo operation.

No magician works without a stage crew.

That's where the media comes in.

You think journalists are curious?

They used to be.
Now they're stenographers in lab goggles.

We give them a headline:

"New study shows…"

And they copy-paste it like gospel.

No follow-up.
No context.
No question about who funded the study or what data was excluded.

Just:

"Experts say."

And that's all it takes.

Let me explain how this works.

We give you a press release.
We write it in soft, passive language:

"Findings suggest"
"Early data indicates"
"Consistent with prior modeling"

You turn on CNN and see:

"BREAKING: Science Confirms."

By the time it hits your feed, the nuance is gone.
What's left is **compliance-friendly certainty**.

Wrapped in blue checks and NPR voices.

During COVID?

It wasn't science reporting.

It was **pandemic theater review**.

They weren't investigating.
They were **amplifying**.

We told them to smear lab-leak theorists.
They called them racist.

We said: "Don't platform dissent."
They said: "We've updated our misinformation policy."

We needed a firewall between the public and the truth.

And the media built it **voluntarily**.

You want to know the real role of journalists during COVID?

To repeat us louder.

To **shame the uncertain**.

To make sure if you doubted the official story,
you'd feel alone.

Because isolation is more powerful than argument.

And fear of social exile?
That's better than any data point I could ever forge.

They called it "debunking."
What it really was: **disbelief laundering**.

Take a dangerous idea—like, say, "the vaccines don't
stop transmission."

Run it through a fact-check factory.

Add six “context experts” who haven’t seen a patient since 2003.

Label it “Partly False.”

Shadowban. Throttle. De-boost.

Now you’ve got the illusion of truth
and the comfort of consensus.

That’s how you build belief systems without belief.

Want to know the ultimate irony?

The people yelling “Trust the science” the loudest?

Didn’t read the science.

They read **the summary of the press release** of the preprint
about the study
written by the graduate assistant
of the PI
who was cashing a Pfizer subgrant.

Then they posted it on Twitter with the caption:

“This you?”

A lot of what I did, I did through the media.

Because **we didn’t need to silence everyone**.

Just enough of them to make the rest look crazy.

That’s not censorship.

That's **infection control**.

And they were **happy to help**.

Let me put it another way:

We didn't need to tell the truth.

We just needed to own the channels people trusted to hear it.

We used to call it "public health communications."

Now we call it what it is:
Narrative engineering.

You've heard of the **military-industrial complex**?

Well this was the **censorship-industrial complex**.

NIH funds the research.
CDC issues the line.
The New York Times prints the line.
Twitter enforces the line.
Facebook algorithmically repeats the line.
Google buries anything that contradicts the line.

And you?

You call that "consensus."

Cute.

We didn't need to bribe the media.
We just needed to give them a **moral framework** and a **feed**.

You give a journalist the illusion that they're fighting fascism and saving Grandma at the same time?

They'll do the propaganda **for free**.

In fact, they'll shame anyone who questions it.

They'll beg for more censorship.

They'll go on Substack witch-hunts and call it "fact-checking."

They'll unfriend their own parents because **Anderson Cooper said so**.

And when someone like Joe Rogan or Bret Weinstein or RFK Jr. started asking real questions?

We didn't need to debate them.

We just *classified* them.

"Dangerous."

"Anti-vax."

"Far-right."

"Russian-adjacent." (Always a crowd favorite.)

Suddenly no one's listening to what they're saying.
They're defending *why* they're allowed to speak.

And once you have to explain yourself?

You've already lost.

Here's how we sold the silence:

"You wouldn't want someone shouting fire in a crowded theater."

But we were the ones **lighting the matches**.

And the people screaming "fire"?
They were trying to **get you out**.

Want to know how far it went?

At one point, **we coordinated with Spotify**.
Yes—Spotify.
The place where you listen to Coldplay and murder podcasts.

Because "science" had to be protected…
on a streaming app.

Because God forbid someone hears **two conflicting viewpoints** and uses their brain.

That's not public health.

That's **unauthorized thinking**.

And let's talk about "disinformation."

It used to mean:

"A provably false statement intended to deceive."

Now?

It means:

"Something true said at the wrong time, by the wrong person, that makes the wrong people uncomfortable."

We didn't just fight a virus.

We fought **unauthorized observation**.

We fought **uncurated awareness**.

We fought **things we couldn't control**—so we labeled them dangerous.

And you believed us.

Not because we were right.

But because **everyone who said otherwise got disappeared**.

That's not a debate.
That's **asymmetrical warfare**.

And we won.

Everything I did, I did with a coalition of the willing:

- Virologists who needed the grant money.
- Journalists who needed the clicks.
- Platforms who feared the Hill.
- And true believers who needed the dopamine of certainty.

We didn't kill science.

We made it **profitable**.

Then we turned it into a brand. Let's talk about the journals.

Because the phrase **"published in a top journal"** used to mean something.

Now?

It means *somebody's budget just cleared.*

Let me tell you how it works.

You do a study. It gets submitted.

The editors send it out for "peer review." That sounds rigorous. You picture a circle of Gandalf-looking experts hurling lightning bolts at bad data.

What's actually happening?

Your reviewer is a postdoc at Stanford who hasn't slept in three days, owes your PI a favor, and clicks "Accept with Minor Revisions" because he's behind on grading.

Or worse:
He's your **co-author from a previous paper**, reviewing you under a different name.

Yes, that happens. A lot.
And if your study finds something… inconvenient?

Say, early treatment works.
Or natural immunity's stronger.
Or vaccines have a side effect window longer than we told you?

Rejected.

Or better—"desk rejected," which means no reviewer ever even saw it.

Then the editor emails you something like:

"Not aligned with our editorial priorities."

Translation:
We don't publish that kind of truth here.

Now flip it around.

You run a half-baked model out of Imperial College predicting 2 million deaths by Christmas?

Fast-tracked.

You plug a dataset into machine learning that spits out "masks reduce transmission by 1.4% in Bangladesh"?

Welcome to *Science*.

You ghostwrite a piece for Pfizer that says the fourth dose boosts antibody levels—without mentioning it was only tested on eight mice?

Nature would like to speak with you. Why?

Because journals aren't independent.
They're **trophy cases for power**.

You think *The Lancet* published Daszak's letter because it was true?

No.

They published it because it was **useful**.

It was cover.

It was an ad wrapped in an exorcism:

"Lab leak theories are dangerous. Trust the experts."

27 signatures.
None of those people disclosed conflicts.
One ghostwrote the damn thing.

And it worked.

Meanwhile, **preprints** became a battlefield.

That's where the inconvenient data lived—briefly.

Then the "fact-checkers" showed up.

Oh yes.
Let's talk about them.

Fact-checking isn't truth-seeking.
It's **narrative restoration**.

A dangerous idea gains traction?

You don't disprove it.

You **flag it**, **contextualize it**, **shadowban it**.

Then you paste a gray box on the screen that says:

"Missing context. See what the WHO says."

That's not critical thinking.

That's **soft policing**.

And it worked on you.

And what about those tech CEOs?

Don't kid yourself.

They didn't want to censor anyone.

But you threaten their liability under Section 230?

Suddenly Facebook becomes a virus information bureau.
YouTube starts deleting Nobel Prize winners.
Twitter bans a Stanford epidemiologist for saying the curve already flattened.

What changed?

We walked into their offices with a folder labeled:

"Misinformation is a public health crisis."

They asked how to help.

We gave them a list.

And then you ask me why nobody knew the truth?

Because **we tied it to a cinder block and threw it in the algorithm**.

And I didn't do it alone.

I did it with partners.

With **funders**, **platforms**, **and "experts"** who understood the same thing I did:

"Reality is not what's provable.
Reality is what's survivable."

And we made it through.

We kept the story alive long enough to bury the evidence under **outrage fatigue**.

Let me explain.

We used to have a clean system.

Science said something.
Journals printed it.
The media echoed it.
You believed it.

Done.

But then… came the **platforms**.

And suddenly?

Everyone had a mic.

Even the people we weren't done discrediting yet.

Even the people we hadn't written counter-narratives for yet.

Even the ones who, God help us, were *actually right*.

The algorithm didn't care about our credentials.

It didn't care about "The Science™."

It just wanted engagement.

And guess what people engage with?

Doubt.

Especially when it sounds **coherent**.

We said:

"Stay inside."

They posted:

"Vitamin D reduces mortality."

We said:

"Get the shot."

They asked:

"Why is myocarditis spiking in teen boys?"

We said:

"Trust the experts."

They asked:

"Then why did the experts lie about masks, lockdowns, natural immunity, the origin?"

And the algorithm?

Boosted them.

Because people clicked.

Because **it felt true**.

So what did we do?

We panicked.

We called the tech companies.

We labeled it all **"misinformation."**

Then we built **a second lab**.

This one in Silicon Valley.

This one to engineer perception the way we used to engineer spike proteins.

We called it **"content moderation."**

But what we were really doing?

PCR testing for narrative loyalty.

And anyone who didn't hit the cycle threshold?

Deleted.

We didn't shut down dissent.

We **mutated it**.

We changed its shape.

Made it harder to find.
Made it seem fringe.
Made it feel exhausting.

You scroll and scroll and scroll…

And all you see is the same thing, slightly rearranged:

"The vaccines are safe."
"COVID is deadly."
"Anyone who disagrees is a threat."

That's not science.

That's **viral load management**.

You're not just misinformed.

You've been **trained** to need permission to believe what's in front of your own damn face.

And guess what?

You're welcome.

Because I'm the one telling you this now.

Why?

Because somebody had to.

If I let it rot quietly—
if I vanished with a pension on a never-ending vacation to Sicily—
then **all the other rats go down with the ship**.

But now?

Now they see the path.

I'm lighting the way out.

Not for you.

For them.

You?

You're on your own.

But the people who helped build this?

The grant writers, the ghost authors, the junior lab assistants who knew what was in the freezer?

They needed a model.

A blueprint for **strategic evacuation**.

And this—this confession? This is it.

Whatever you think I did —and yes, I did it—
you should thank me.

Because without me saying it out loud,
you'd still be praying to "the science"
while the hull fills with water
and the band plays you off the edge.

I got out first.

Now they know how to follow.

That's leadership.

That's legacy. That's **ethics**, baby.

CHAPTER 14

Event 201

The Rehearsal We Weren't Supposed to Talk About

Everyone keeps bringing up **Event 201**, like it's some kind of smoking gun.

"October 2019."
"Pandemic simulation."
"Funded by Gates and the World Economic Forum."
"Three months before Wuhan."

Yes.
All of that is true.

We did it.
We ran the simulation.
We gamed out what would happen if a novel coronavirus broke out and circled the globe.

And you know what?

It went almost exactly like the real thing.

I know how that sounds.

Like we planned it.
Like the virus was queued up backstage while we practiced the messaging.

But that's not how it happened. For that you'll have to read to the end.

Event 201 wasn't the plot.
It was the **blueprint**.

A fire drill.

But the kind where the fire breaks out during the exercise—
and everyone decides not to tell the public that the smoke is real.
Here's the thing:

The people in that room?
They weren't amateurs.

- CIA.
- CDC.
- Johns Hopkins.
- The Gates Foundation.
- The UN.
- World Bank.
- Corporate media reps and pharmaceutical liaisons.

Not crackpots.
Not prepper weirdos.
Professionals.

And what we practiced wasn't science.
It was **messaging**.

How to control the narrative.
How to "pre-bunk" dissent.
How to frame skepticism as a threat to public health.
How to partner with media and tech platforms to **shape the signal**.

We didn't focus on ventilators.
We focused on **compliance**.

And that's why it worked.

So yes—we walked through a coronavirus outbreak just **weeks before** one emerged.

We discussed:

- Censorship coordination
- Government-corporate "information alignment"
- Suppressing rumors that questioned the origin of the pathogen
- Pushing unified vaccine messaging
- Managing economic fallout with strategic communications

And when the real virus showed up?

We **used the same playbook**.

Because it was already laminated.

Was it coincidence?

Maybe.

But let me ask you:

When a group of military contractors runs a nuclear strike simulation—and then a missile actually launches the next month—

Do you call that a coincidence?

Or do you call it **familiarity with the terrain**?

Let's back up.

October 18, 2019.
New York City.
The simulation was hosted by:

- **The Johns Hopkins Center for Health Security**
- **The Bill & Melinda Gates Foundation**
- **The World Economic Forum**

The scenario?
A novel coronavirus spills over from bats to humans,
spreads globally through air travel,
and overwhelms health systems while panic and disinformation threaten social cohesion.

It sounds familiar because it is.

We didn't imagine the future.

We **rehearsed** it.

It wasn't a science roundtable.

It was a **command-and-control war game**.

No time was spent modeling cytokine storms or mutational drift. We weren't reviewing trial protocols or outbreak response logistics.

We were running **narrative containment simulations**.

The goal wasn't stopping the virus.
It was stopping the **wrong interpretation** of the virus.

We discussed:

- How to "pre-bunk" theories about lab origins before they spread
- Which media outlets would partner on "information campaigns"
- How to suppress dissent "without appearing authoritarian"
- How to manage "reluctant" populations during mass vaccination efforts
- What kind of financial levers could be pulled to incentivize compliance
- How to coordinate talking points across international bodies

We even role-played government officials getting grilled for slow response times— and how to **pivot the blame** to citizens, misinformation, and budget cuts.

In short:
We practiced managing perception, not pandemic.

And it was **designed to keep people in line**.

The masks.
The distancing.
The media partnerships.
The daily death trackers.
The disinformation task forces.

Not improvised.
Not grassroots.

Scripted.

And that plan didn't center on truth.
It centered on **control**.

Because by 2019, we'd learned something:

You can't manage biology.
You can only manage **belief**.

So yes—Event 201 happened.

And yes—we were proud of how it went.

And when the real thing arrived?

We didn't go back to the whiteboard.

We **hit "Print."**

Event 201 was the first draft.

The pandemic was just the final production.

And you?

You weren’t the audience.

You were the test subject.

CHAPTER 15

The Needle and the Lie

I Turn My Scalpel on the Vaccine Industrial Complex I Helped Build

You're Welcome for the Injections

You want to talk about vaccines?

Fine.

Let's talk about **what they actually are now**.

Because what you think they are—
and what they've become?

Those are two different compounds entirely.

You think "vaccine" means a weakened virus.
Something that triggers immunity.
A noble shield.
A miracle.
A memory from childhood.

But that's ***the old model***.
That's ***rotary club logic***.

Little paper sugar cubes and Eisenhower smiles.

The new model?

Is code.

Today's vaccines don't introduce viruses.

They introduce ***instructions***.

Synthetic sequences.
Wrapped in lipid envelopes.

Delivered by needle.
Expressed in ***your*** cells.

We tell your body to build the thing it's supposed to be afraid of.

Then we watch what happens.

That's not immunology.

That's ***programming***.

And you?

You let us do it.

Because we called it **protection**.

And when people asked questions?

We called them ***dangerous***.

Let's go back to ***SV40***.

Simian Virus 40.

You didn't hear about it in school.

You should've.

Because it was ***the first real tell***.

Late 1950s.

The world's in a panic about ***polio***.

Children in iron lungs.
Wheelchairs.
March of Dimes.
Dr. Salk becomes a saint.

We rush the vaccine.

We scale production using **monkey kidney cells**.

Because that's what we had.

What we didn't realize?

Those monkeys were ***carrying a virus***.

SV40.

Undetected.
Unfiltered.
Unmentioned.

It ended up in ***over 90 million doses***.

Injected.
Swallowed.
Mass distributed.

The CDC knew.

The NIH knew.

Eventually ***everybody knew***.

But it was ***too late***.

And the optics? Unacceptable.

So what did we do?

Simple:

"There's no conclusive evidence SV40 causes cancer in humans."

Case closed.

Except it **does** cause cancer.

In ***rats***.

In ***hamsters***.

In ***every model we tested it in***.

It integrates into DNA.
It disrupts ***tumor suppressor genes***.

It lingers.
It replicates.
It leaves ***nothing but deniability***.

You ask me:

"How did we let that happen?"

We didn't "let it happen."

We ***needed*** it to happen.

Because the ***production pipeline*** was the real breakthrough.

Not the vaccine.

The ***system***.

The scale.

The ***ability to inject millions before asking what's inside***.

SV40 was our first ***vaccine-borne contaminant***.

It wasn't the last.

But it was the one that taught us the golden rule:

**If the public is scared enough,
you can put anything in their arm.**

Saint Bill and the Salvation Supply Chain

Let's talk about ***Bill***.

Yes, that Bill.

Windows Bill.
CTRL+ALT+DEL Bill.
Monopoly trials and smirk-in-a-sweater Bill.

He left the software world and ***decided to fix the real one***.

And what did he choose?

Not sanitation.
Not housing.
Not nutrition.

Vaccines.

Because vaccines are **clean**.
Scalable.
Traceable.
And ***profitable—even when they're not***.

He didn't just donate money.

He built ***an ecosystem***.

He gave the world ***GAVI***.

The Vaccine Alliance.

Sounds like a Marvel team.

It's not.

It's ***a distribution cartel with nonprofit branding***.

GAVI isn't in the science business.

It's in the ***last-mile enforcement business***.

Their job?

Make sure the vaccine ***gets into arms***—

Not because of disease burden.

Because ***that's the product***.

Bill figured out early what SV40 had already proven:

"You don't need a perfect vaccine.
You need a ***global delivery system***
with no refund policy."

So that's what he built. Here's the playbook:

- Set up a foundation.
- Fund the WHO.
- Partner with pharma.
- Subsidize deployment through GAVI.
- Leverage media to moralize uptake.

- Dismiss criticism as anti-science.
- Repeat.

You think you're protecting children?

You're ***executing logistics***.

Gates didn't just fund vaccines.

He ***deputized the concept***.

He made vaccination ***a moral absolute***.

Question it?

You're a threat to humanity.

Not just ***wrong***.
Dangerous.

That's how you control the debate.

You don't argue.

You ***elevate the baseline***.

And don't forget:

He doesn't need to mandate anything.

Because GAVI ***ties access to compliance***.

Want school?

Shot.

Want food aid?

Shot.

Want to get on the plane?

Show us ***your updated QR code***.

The Virus Left—But We Still Had Syringes to Fill

Once upon a time, a vaccine was a virus.

Attenuated.
Weakened.
Sometimes killed.
Still recognizable.
Still dangerous.
Still real.

The immune system saw it and said: "I know you."

That was enough.

Then came the pivot.

We stopped using viruses.

Why?

- Too slow.
- Too dirty.

- Too many lab mishaps.
- Too much paperwork.

So we switched to ***components***.

Fragments.
Vectors.
Nucleic acid codes.
Synthetic instructions.

But here's the thing:

Your immune system's not impressed by ***instructions***.

It doesn't see code and panic.

It sees ***nothing***.

So we had to **spike the punch**.

We needed ***adjuvants***.

You've heard the word.

You probably never asked what it meant.

Adjuvants are ***immune irritants***.

They don't teach the body to recognize a threat.

They ***trick it into reacting***.

Like setting off a fire alarm during a drill.

Just to make sure ***somebody*** notices.

The early adjuvants were simple:

- **Aluminum salts.**
  Cheap. Aggressive. Long-lasting.
  Still used.

But newer ones?

- ***Squalene emulsions***
- ***TLR agonists***
- ***Polysorbate-80 blends***
- ***Nanoparticle-stabilized mRNA vesicles***

You don't know what those are.

That's the point.

We say ***"safe and effective."***

You hear ***"vaccine."***

You don't ask ***what else is in the vial.***

And that's where things get tricky.

Because adjuvants ***don't always shut off.***

They spark inflammation.
They **override tolerance thresholds.**
They sometimes ***stick around.***

Long after the antigen's gone.

You think the side effects came from the spike protein?

Sometimes, yes.

But a lot of it?

***Came from the ignition system*.**

The ***flame, not the fuel*.**

Why didn't we tell you?

Because ***the platform matters more than the payload*.**

Once we had ***proof of concept*—**
"Look! It produces antibodies!"—

We stopped asking ***what else it does*.**

Especially long-term.

Especially ***in complex human bodies*** with ***different genetic baselines*.**

Nonprofit Means Never Having to Say What You're Testing

You see the word "nonprofit"
and your brain shuts off.

"They're helping."

"They care."

"They're not in it for the money."

Cute.

Let me tell you what nonprofit means in the global vaccine world:

No liability.
No transparency.
No brakes.

Start with ***GAVI.***

We already talked about it.

The delivery arm.

The lockstep mechanism that ensures ***nobody slips through the injection net.***

Then there's ***CEPI.***

Coalition for Epidemic Preparedness Innovations.

Sounds like a UN offshoot.

It's ***a research slush fund.***

mRNA at warp speed.
Novel adjuvants.
Pre-pandemic production pipelines.

They don't ask if it's needed.

They ask ***if it's fundable.***

Then there's ***PATH.***

They operate in Asia and Africa mostly.

Smiling brochures.
Community health workers.
Cold chain pilots.

They say they're advancing health equity.

What they're actually doing?

Real-time field deployment studies.

Behavioral feedback loops.

Uptake experiments.

Biometric ID integration.

Ever wonder why ***the Gates Foundation*** funds ***both*** the trial
and the NGO delivering it
and the WHO guideline that follows?

That's not charity.

That's ***vertical integration***.

Here's the genius:

When a pharma company tests a vaccine?

You get headlines.
Lawsuits.
Pushback.

When a ***nonprofit*** rolls it out?

You get ***Nobel nominations***.

And the testing?

Doesn't happen in New York.

It happens in ***villages***.

Low-data environments.
Minimal reporting.
No lawyers.
No media.
Just ***checkpoints and promises***.

You want to know how we field-tested ***multi-dose mRNA programs***?

GAVI in Uganda.

You want to know how we rolled out ***QR-based vax credentials***?

India's Aadhaar-linked pilot program.

You want to know how we trialed ***combined shot + social service programs***?

Gates-funded women's clinics in Bangladesh.

And the best part?

It's ***all opt-in***.

Until it's not.

"The Empire Wore a Lab Coat"

You think governments ran the pandemic?

No.

Governments ***responded***.

The ones who ran it?

Didn't wear flags.

They wore ***foundation logos***.

Start with ***Gates***.

Already covered him.
But remember—he doesn't just fund GAVI.

He funds:

- The WHO
- CEPI
- Johns Hopkins
- Oxford
- Imperial College
- The *Washington Post*
- Global health "task forces"
- Media "misinformation" monitors
- And ***his own reporting on all of it***.

That's ***vertical integration***.

That's ***god mode***.

Then there's ***The Wellcome Trust***.

Quiet.

Old money.

Tied to ***GlaxoSmithKline***.

They call themselves ***independent***.

They're not.

They fund ***narrative studies***.
Behavioral research.
Health equity work.

Which means?

They write the moral script.

And the media ***reads from it***.

Rockefeller Foundation?
Still alive.
Still shaping vaccine financing.
Still writing "resilience playbooks."
Still pushing ***biosurveillance infrastructure*** in the name of justice.

You know what that means?

"We're going to scan you.
Forever.
Because fairness."

Then there's ***Clinton Health Access Initiative***.

Sounds like a nonprofit.

It's ***a rollout arm***.

They negotiate vaccine pricing.
They structure deals.
They tie shots to ***service access in developing regions***.

You want healthcare?

You get ***the shot first***.

That's not medicine.

That's ***soft leverage***.

This wasn't charity.

It was ***market expansion wrapped in empathy***.

The goal?

Simple.

- Get the world used to ***ID-linked injections***.
- Build ***distribution networks***.
- Partner with ***corporate logistics***.
- Fund ***the narrative***.
- Normalize ***the dependency***.

And most of all?

Be untouchable.

Because when you wear a suit?

You can be questioned.

When you wear a ***foundation badge***?

You're ***above scrutiny***.

"Just trying to help."

That's the final shield.

That's ***the final lab coat***.

I didn't build the empire.

I just ***wore the crest on camera***.

And when it was time to fall?

They were already ***on to the next crisis***.

Smiling.

Sanitized.

And ***still tax-exempt***.

CHAPTER 16

The Spreadsheet People Ruined Everything

I thought we could bury it in boilerplate.
PDFs. Dashboards. Jargon.
We wrapped the truth in Helvetica and hoped no one zoomed in.
And for a while, no one did.
But I forgot about ***the spreadsheet people***.

It started with a mom.
No credentials. No press pass.
Just a dead kid, a wi-fi connection, and an Excel filter.
She saw the pattern in ER visits.
Connected it to batch numbers.
Posted it.
Then others joined.
Not scientists. Not journalists.
Just people who still knew how to read before they were told what it meant. We couldn't stop them.

They weren't journalists.
They weren't activists.
They weren't even on Twitter half the time.

They were ***freaks with bar graphs***.

And they ***never needed us***.

By the way, it wasn't a journalist who caught me.
It was a mom.
In a kitchen.
Color-coding a Google Sheet while the baby napped.
And when people started listening to her?
The game was over.
Sourced.

And ***backed up in six places***.

There's one kind of person I'll never win against.

It's not a politician.
It's not a journalist.
It's ***a mom with a spreadsheet and a dead kid***.

I can bury data.
I can spin trials.
I can throttle articles.
But I can't ***out-stubborn grief***.

Especially when it's ***righteous***.

Especially when it's ***organized***.

And now?

They've gone from angry to ***fluent***.

They can quote VAERS data better than ***my staff***.

They know ***dose schedules, formulation changes, adjuvant patents, legislative history***.

They know ***which CDC meetings were quietly canceled***.

They even know ***how to pronounce aluminum hydroxide***.

And they're not doing it for clout.

They're not doing it for grants.

They're doing it because ***we messed with their kids***.

We gave ***a hepatitis B vaccine*** to ***newborns***.

Within 24 hours of birth.

You know how you get Hep B?

Needles or sex.

Explain that to a mother holding a six-pound baby in a bassinet under blue light.

Go ahead.

I couldn't.

But I approved it.

Why?

Because ***we wanted the market***.

And because ***we had the protection***.

Ever heard of the ***National Childhood Vaccine Injury Act of 1986***?

Passed it after ***a few kids died***.
The industry was ***about to collapse under liability***.

So we made a deal.

- No lawsuits.
- No courtrooms.
- Just ***a special tribunal***.
- Funded by ***you***.

You pay a tax on every shot.

That funds the payout pool.

If your kid dies?

You file a claim.

If you're lucky, ***you get a check***.

If not?

Too bad.

Either way?

There's less than a 0.1% chance you ever see a dime.

That's when things really took off.

After 1986?

The childhood schedule exploded.

Before: ~10 shots.

Now?

Upwards of ***72 doses before age 18***.

All protected.

All ***marketed as required***.

All ***bundled into pediatric care***.

You want school? You want daycare? You want peace?

Roll up the baby's sleeve.

And when people asked:

"Why so many?" We said:

"Trust the experts."

But we never explained ***the structure we were protecting***.

Because the structure ***was the goal***.

I didn't underestimate these people asking questions.

I ***hoped they'd give up***.

But they didn't.

Because ***they're not fighting to win Twitter***.

They're fighting because ***we lied where it hurts most***.

And ***they don't get tired***.

The Story Slipped Out of My Hands

There's a moment every storyteller fears.

It's not when you're challenged.

It's when ***you're no longer the narrator***.

I could feel it shift.

Subtle at first.

People weren't ***waiting*** for the *New York Times*.

They weren't ***retweeting*** **Nature**.

They weren't ***repeating me***.

They were ***talking to each other***.

Telegram groups.
Homeschooling networks.
Substacks with ***more citations than we ever used internally***.

People ***cross-checking lot numbers***.

People ***mapping injury clusters***.

People r***ecording their own family histories—***
in public.

And ***other people listening***.

They stopped asking:

"What does Fauci think?"

And started asking:

"What happened to my neighbor?"

"Why did my healthy friend collapse?"

"Why are all these pilots getting grounded?"

"Why did my kid's school suddenly have a defibrillator?"

That wasn't press failure.

That was ***press irrelevance***.

Because once the personal outnumbers the official?

The narrative's gone.

It belongs to ***the crowd now***.

And the crowd ***remembers differently***.

They remember ***the gaslighting***.

They remember ***the masking contradictions***.

They remember ***the side effects brushed off.***

They remember ***the way we mocked them for noticing.***

And they ***don't need CNN to tell them how they feel.***

They ***already know.***

We thought we could outlast it.

We thought people would forget.

We ***built the whole system on that hope.***

But they didn't.

And now?

The narrative is ***happening without us.***

It's ***organic.***
Uncontrolled.
Permanent.

I didn't lose control because of a scandal.

I lost it because ***the people started talking.***

And ***listening to each other.***

And when that happens?

You ***can't put the story back in the syringe.***

We always feared ***a congressional inquiry.***

A scandal.

A leaker.

A smoking gun.

We were prepared for that.

We had ***talking points***.

We had ***cutouts***.

We had ***plausible deniability filed in triplicate***.

But that's not what happened.

What happened was ***quieter***.

And ***worse***.

People just ***started walking away***.

Not with torches.

Not with lawsuits.

With ***resignation***.

With ***closed laptops***.

With ***"no, thank you."***

Doctors ***stopped recommending***.
Nurses ***stopped asking***.
Parents ***stopped complying***.
Pharmacists ***stopped ordering***.
Journalists ***stopped calling***.

Not because they flipped.

Because they ***figured it out***.

They ***didn't need proof***.

They ***lived it***.

They ***watched it happen***.
To friends.
To coworkers.
To ***their own kids***.

And once that happens?

Trust doesn't come back.

We thought ***the fear would hold***.

We built ***systems around that***.

Vaccine passports.
Employer mandates.
College boosters.

But fear has a half-life.

And when it decays?

All that's left is ***memory***.

And ***rage***.

Now?

The clinics are empty.
The uptake charts are flatlining.
The ad campaigns are pathetic.
The budgets are bloated and ***nobody's showing up***.

We burned ***decades of trust*** in ***two years***.

And we have ***no plan for what to do when no one believes us again***.

This wasn't ***a rebellion***.

It was ***a slow exodus***.

And it's still happening.

I didn't trigger the reckoning.

I just ***set the conditions for one***.

And it ***didn't knock on the front door***.

It ***walked out the back***.

One person at a time.

Without a sound.

I still get invites.

Panels.
Lectures.
Closed-door "resilience summits."

The same people.
The same language.
The same acronyms.

But something's different.

There's ***no audience***.

The press releases go out.

No one picks them up.

The studies get published.

No one reads them.

The funding rolls in.

But ***the faith is gone***.

I scroll through inboxes.

Old contacts.
Old journalists.
Old allies.

The ones who used to forward every op-ed, every hit piece, every "debunking."

Now?

Unread.

Or worse—

"Unsubscribed."

We didn't just lose the public.

We lost ***the middle***.

The teachers.
The nurses.
The normies.
The guy who used to say, "Well, the CDC says—"

Now ***he doesn't***.

Now ***he doesn't say anything at all***.

That's how systems end.

Not with fire.

With ***silence***.

With ***ghost town waiting rooms***.

With ***epidemiologists tweeting into the void***.

With ***public health announcements nobody hears***.

The machine's still humming.

The emails still go out.

The committees still meet.

But ***the story's over***.

And ***I can't tell it again***.

Because ***no one's listening***.

I'm not the one who destroyed the trust.

I ***overdrew it***.

And now ***the account is closed***.

Permanently.

CHAPTER 17

The Transfer

They thought Warp Speed was about vaccines.
It wasn't.

They thought it was about science.
Nope.

It was about **control**.
About *proving* something.
About showing the world—
and more importantly, the bureaucracy—
that we could move faster
than the government
if we just cut the government out of the way.

Let me back up.

We had a problem.
A big one.
Not the virus.
Not the deaths.
Not the confusion.

The problem was this:
Elected officials were still pretending to be in charge.

That had to end.

So we gave them Warp Speed.
A miracle with a deadline.
The illusion of urgency.
Wrapped in flag colors.
Backed by generals.

It looked like a Trump thing.
It felt like a moon landing.
But behind the curtain?

We were rearranging the furniture.

No more HHS bottlenecks.
No more agency silos.
We had inter-agency override.
We had DOD logistics.
We had pre-approved pathways.

We rewrote procurement protocols in real time.
We **overrode Congressional purse strings** by calling it war.
And no one blinked.

Because everyone wanted the cure.
No one read the contract.

We built the machine.
They pushed the button.
And the beauty of it was—
they thought it was theirs.

Trump called it his Apollo program.
Biden called it a miracle of science.

We called it
the acceleration of permanent authority.

The vaccine wasn't the point.

The point was:
we created a precedent.

An expectation.

A new operating model.
Where elected leaders stand at the podium—
but **we write the slides**.

They never got it.
Not Trump.
Not Biden.

They took credit for the rollout.
We took custody of the infrastructure.

Now?
We have platforms.
We have standing funding.
We have agile authorizations that bypass the old chains.

And no one's clawing it back.
Not Congress.
Not the courts.
Not the public.

Because we saved lives.
And you can get away with anything
if you say it saved lives.

You want to know what Warp Speed really did?

It proved
we don't need permission anymore.

It taught a generation of staffers
that we can move billions
with a declaration and a task force.

It showed career officials
how to **survive a rotating presidency**
by building systems that outlive elections.

It replaced ceremony with continuity.
And continuity
always wins.

Look, I'll say it:
Presidents are loud.
We're quiet.

They tweet.
We draft.

They vanish.
We remain.

Warp Speed was never about ending COVID.
It was about **what came after**.

Emergency use.
Central supply chains.
Data capture.
Federalized health authority.
No debate. **No delay**. **No vote**.

That's what stayed.
That's what mattered.

So yes—
the shots went out.
People clapped.
And presidents took bows.

But behind the velvet rope?
We upgraded the system.

We made ourselves
indispensable.

And that, my friend,
is the real cure.

CHAPTER 18

The Cure Performed Worse Than the Disease

Let's stop pretending.

We didn't just fail.

We made it ***worse***.

Start with the scoreboard: **All-cause mortality**.

The one number we couldn't spin.

You want to know how it looked in the U.S.?

Up.

After the vaccine rollout.

Not during Delta.
Not during Alpha.
After.

Heart attacks.
Strokes.
Sudden deaths.
Turbo cancers.
Neuro weirdness.

We didn't need whistleblowers.

The insurance companies told the truth by accident.

"Something's off."

Yeah.

That was ***us***.

Other countries?

Same trend.

But the worse the outcomes?

The ***more vaxxed they were***.

Israel.
Scotland.
New Zealand.
Canada.
The U.K.

It wasn't just correlation.

It was ***a pattern we couldn't admit***.

Because the product was still live.

We told you:

"It will end the pandemic."

What it ended was ***the illusion of control.***

And ***public trust***.

And then?

Trump won again.

Not officially.

But ***culturally***.

The institutions we propped up with science?

They cracked.

People didn't come back to CNN.

They went ***full MAHA***.

Make America Healthy Again.

And ***RFK***?

Not outside the system.

He's inside the courtroom.

You know what happens when someone who's ***been reading footnotes since 2003*** finally gets subpoena power?

We ***panic***.

We ***reformat laptops***.

We ***microwave hard drives***.

I've seen it.

Every agency has a drawer full of ***"broken backups."***

And the ones that aren't broken?

Might be tomorrow.

You think I stayed because I loved the camera?

You think I needed the attention?

Let me clear that up.

I stayed because ***if I stopped talking,***
they'd start asking questions.

The wrong ones.

As long as I was **Director of NIAID**,
as long as I had a government badge,
as long as ***I was essential***,

I wasn't a civilian.

And that meant:

- No direct subpoenas.
- No leak liability.

- No retroactive culpability for ***what I signed, approved, or buried***.

I had ***classified clearance***.

I had ***press armor***.

I had ***plausible deniability built into the org chart***.

But the moment I left?

I became ***just another guy with a pension and a paper trail***.

And I knew the paper trail was **getting warm**.

RFK was climbing in the polls.

Trump was winning counties with ***vaccine injury town halls***.

MAHA moms were walking into public comment sessions ***with spreadsheets and death certificates***.

And ***journalists we couldn't buy*** started asking questions ***we didn't prepare answers for***.

Inside the agencies? The tone changed.

People ***stopped replying to emails***.

Calendars went ***blank***.

Everyone started ***checking old Dropbox folders to see what needed deleting***.

And when that wasn't enough?

We bought microwaves.

Actual microwaves.

Not for lunch.

For ***flash formatting backup drives.***

That's when I knew:

I couldn't leave.

Not yet.

Not until ***we had a fall guy lined up.***

Not until ***the chain of custody got fuzzy enough to blame an intern or a dead guy.***

Not until ***the hard questions had new names in the cc field.***

Because once I left?

Once I became ***Dr. Fauci, private citizen***?

Goodbye ***protection.***

No briefings.

No immunity.

No backchannel to call the editor.

Just ***me***.

And ***the ghosts I helped make***.

CHAPTER 19

The Early Days (or Why I Can't Say No Now)

People think the blackmail started with Wuhan.
Wrong.

If anyone's got leverage on me, it didn't come from bats.
It came from **decades of doing what needed to be done**—and making deals to keep the machine running.

Because that's the thing about long careers:
You survive by **saying yes to things you pretend not to remember**.
I came up through NIH in the post-AIDS chaos.
Back when science wasn't polished.
Back when data got buried, side effects got minimized, and patients learned about trial failures from **obituaries**, not journal articles.

I was there when **AZT** was pushed through.
I was there when we told the public it was safe—knowing full well the dose was crushing people's bone marrow.

We called it "urgency."
We said the risk was worth it.
And maybe it was.

But we never looked back.
Not publicly.

And that became the model.

Every time there was a crisis, we got more powerful.

- Anthrax? We expanded biodefense funding by billions.
- SARS-1? We rewrote how trials were run.
- Ebola? We cut corners on protocols—then called it innovation.
- Zika? We scared the hell out of pregnant women and moved mRNA into human testing.

Each time, we pushed further.
Faster.
Looser.

And with every exception we made, we gave someone leverage.

You think China doesn't know what we approved under the table?

You think EcoHealth didn't keep receipts?
You think Baric didn't run side projects no one ever audited?

Hell, even **within NIH**, there are people who know things.
Grants that got waved through.
Reviews that never happened.
Emails that were "deleted" but archived elsewhere.

And the private sector?

They've got everything.
Pharma never forgets who moved a trial forward six months early.
Or who cleared a liability exemption just in time for a rollout.

You think I don't get reminded of that?
I get *very polite emails.*

So yeah—maybe I've lied by omission.

But omission's just another word for **debt management**.

When you know too much, and too many people owe you—or could sink you—you learn to walk carefully.

Say enough to stay credible. Not enough to get erased.

And if someone whispers "DEFUSE" in a meeting?
You nod.
And you change the subject.

If I'm compromised, it didn't start with Wuhan.

It started the first time I let a drug through without enough data.
The first time I said, "*We'll fix the adverse effects later.*"
The first time I let a contractor write their own results summary.

Those things stack up.

And eventually?

They build a wall behind you.

So when the call comes—
when someone says, *"You're going to help us manage this narrative"*—

You don't argue.

You already used up your "No."

CHAPTER 20

The Leak Before the Leak

If You Think COVID Was the Crime, You Still Don't Get the Motive

Let's get something straight.

COVID wasn't the real scandal.

It was **the cover-up for the real scandal**.

And the real scandal?

Had feathers.

You remember avian flu, right?

H5N1.
The bird one.
Killed half the people it infected—60% case fatality rate in some clusters.

Didn't spread easily between humans.
But that was just a detail.

A *technicality* we were actively trying to erase in the lab.

We told you we were studying it to "understand transmission."
To "prevent pandemics."

But we weren't preventing anything.

We were **forcing evolution**.

Ralph Baric, Ron Fouchier, Kawaoka—all the usual suspects—were up to their necks in it:

- Airborne transmissibility experiments in ferrets.
- Serial passaging.
- Receptor binding enhancements.
- Mutations we hoped nature *might* produce—so we did it for her.

Because why wait?

Let me hit you with a date:

2011.

Fouchier makes H5N1 go airborne in ferrets.
Publishes it.
Sparks an international firestorm.

"This could kill millions."
"This is illegal."
"This violates the Biological Weapons Convention."

Yeah. We heard all of that.

And we did it anyway.

Then came the 2014 pause.
Obama-era moratorium on gain-of-function for flu, SARS, MERS.

Did we stop?

No.

We **rerouted**.

EcoHealth kept the money flowing.
China kept the work going.
And when we needed cover, we called it **"high-risk pathogen surveillance."**

That's how we moved it forward without technically breaking the rules.

We didn't break the rules.

We changed the labels.

Now here's where it gets cute.

2018–2019.

While DEFUSE is being floated (you remember that one—furin cleavage insertions, pre-pandemic SARS upgrades),
we're also cranking out **avian flu studies** that make the virus more human-compatible.

Yeah.

Let me repeat that:

While everyone was focused on bat coronaviruses, we were **tuning up the one that kills 6 out of 10 people**.

We even published it in *Nature*.

Because nothing says "we're totally innocent" like peer-reviewed proof you made a bioweapon with a higher kill rate than COVID.

And then?

It goes quiet.

Mid-to-late 2019:

- WHO flu surveillance reports suddenly dry up.
- Whispers about lab incidents.
- Dead researchers.
- Unexplained pneumonia.
- U.S. intel warning about "an incident" in Wuhan—but no one says what kind.

And then…

COVID.

The magic trick.
The floodlight so bright it obscured the blood spatter behind it.

That's the part they'll never print in *The New York Times*:
COVID didn't just emerge.

It arrived on cue.

Right when the avian flu program was on the edge of exposure.

Right when **questions** were starting to pile up.

Right when we needed the public to look at one lab and **forget about the other freezer**.

I didn't release COVID.

I released **the story of COVID**.

Because it was easier to explain a once-in-a-century coronavirus than a leaking H5N1 prototype that technically violated every treaty we ever signed.

COVID was the **crash mat**.

The softer landing.

The lesser evil.

The Disappearing Data Trick

By mid-2019, we were in deep.

We had at least **three separate programs** pushing avian flu gain-of-function globally:

1. U.S. Department of Defense funding through **DTRA**
2. NIH/NIAID grants routed through **EcoHealth**
3. And our not-so-beloved friend, **USAID's PREDICT program**—a wildlife sampling front disguised as "global health infrastructure."

And the hub?

Wuhan.

Not just for coronaviruses.

For flu, too.

Yeah.
They don't print that part.

Now here's where it gets **eerily quiet**.

In **July 2019**, just a few months before COVID becomes a headline?

The **WHO FluNet system**—the global database tracking influenza surveillance—starts going dark in key regions.

Fewer samples.
Missing sequence updates.
Labs reporting "technical issues."

Then **EcoHealth stops publishing** H5 sequences from their field partners.

Then **PREDICT funding gets quietly pulled** in October.

Almost like **someone was told to shut the tap off**.

We didn't lose surveillance.

We **turned it off**.

And called it… restructuring.

Now ask yourself:

Why do you shut off surveillance **right before** a known pandemic-capable virus family is undergoing aggressive enhancement in at least two labs?

Why does WHO **scrub sequence archives** at the same time researchers are adding mutations to make H5N1 bind to human ACE2 receptors?

Why does the U.S. intel community get **briefed on "unusual lab activity in Wuhan"** in **November 2019**—but everyone thinks it's about a coronavirus?

Because that's the play:

Focus on the right story.
Forget the wrong virus.

This wasn't just scientific curiosity.

This was **intentional escalation**.

2019 was the year we crossed the final line:

We didn't just **enhance H5N1**.

We started teaching it to move like COVID.

Insertions.
Backbone swaps.
Human-cell compatibility tuning.

We didn't just take a deadly virus.

We gave it **ambition**.

So here's the part you're not supposed to ask:

What if something slipped?

Not SARS-CoV-2.
Something else.

Something deadlier.
Shorter incubation.
Harder to trace.

Something that **got loose** in mid to late 2019—
but **burned itself out** before it could make a splash.

What would we do?

Would we admit it?

Would we launch a global investigation?

Or would we—

Drop a different leak.

That's the move, right?

You don't stop the fire.

You **start another one somewhere else**—bigger, flashier, easier to manage.

If H5N1 with human transmission got out,
even just **for a second**,
we'd all be in handcuffs.

No deniability.
No "natural origin" theories.
No pangolins.

But if SARS-CoV-2 appears first?

Suddenly **everything else gets buried**.

All the attention.
All the sequencing teams.
All the FOIA requests.

Diverted.
COVID wasn't the catastrophe.

It was **the cover**.

And the story you've been chasing for four years?

It's the **wrong one**.

The Studies That Went Missing

So. You've got a virus—H5N1—that kills more than half the people it infects.

You've got teams making it more transmissible.

And you've got **papers**—real ones—laying out exactly how they did it:

- Modifying **PB2 gene segments** to enable mammalian adaptation.
- Adding mutations to the **HA receptor binding domain** so it locks onto **alpha-2, 6-linked sialic acids**—the stuff inside your nose.
- Passaging through ferrets to build in stealth.

Each paper is a **manual**.

Each method is a **blueprint**.

And we **published** them.

For "transparency."

For "readiness."

You know—so that **any postdoc with Wi-Fi and a chip on their shoulder** could re-create a weaponized flu strain from a PDF.

Great job, team.

And then… the silence.

Around **Q3 2019**, certain studies start getting **delisted**.

Some never get submitted.
Some die at the preprint level.
Some get "scooped," then vanish.

One particularly spicy Japanese study, which modeled H5N1 adaptation in ferrets using structural modeling + live virus challenge, made it **to peer review**.

Then?
Gone.

Authors ghosted.

Journal retracted the preprint before it hit page one.

Why?

No comment.

But I'll give you mine:

"Too close to what actually happened."

Meanwhile, in the intel world?

We got **cables**.

- October 2019: CDC China field officers recall being denied access to WIV **"due to BSL upgrades."**
- November: DARPA team flagged "abnormal movement" at **two regional flu BSL-3 labs** in Guangdong and Yunnan.
- December: NSA pulls a ***silent ping*** from a private WeChat group among Chinese virologists discussing a "frozen sample breach."

None of this made the timeline.

Not the WHO's.
Not the NIH's.
Not yours.

But I had it.

And so did a few others.

And we agreed—without ever needing to speak—

It's not COVID.
It's something else.

Now imagine you're sitting on all of this.

Imagine you know that a **H5N1-enhanced strain**, one that s*hould not exist*, just **barely brushed against open air**.

Maybe someone got sick.
Maybe a junior lab tech.

Maybe it didn't spread far.

Maybe it did, and we called it "atypical pneumonia" and filed it under "non-COVID viral respiratory infection."

Point is—

You're **this close** to a total unraveling.

So what do you do?

Simple.

You light the flare.

SARS-CoV-2.
Codon-optimized.
Furin cleavage site.
Lateral spread.
Low IFR.
Perfect panic ratio.

Enough to justify lockdowns, EUA, suppression, censorship, consolidation—

But not enough to make people look **past it**.

We didn't just pivot from bird flu.

We ***diluted it***.

We made the world chase a ghost
so it would never find the bones.

The Samples We Kept Moving

Let's talk about the freezer.

Yunnan, southern China.
Dense, wet, viral as hell.
Home to **bat caves, poultry markets, and quiet little labs with no real firewalls**.

We set up operations there years ago.
PREDICT, Metabiota, UC Davis.

All there under the "global biosurveillance" banner.

But let's stop pretending:

It was a **forward operating base**.

A launchpad for the virome gold rush.

From 2009 to 2019, **over 11,000 virus samples** were shipped globally—some straight to Wuhan.
That part you may have read.

What you probably didn't?

Is that ***many of those weren't coronaviruses***.

They were **avian influenzas**.
H5s. H7s.
Highly pathogenic strains, some with internal mutations that made them **ideal templates** for human adaptation studies.

And we didn't stop shipping them just because COVID started trending.

We kept going.

Right into **late 2019, early 2020**.

Yes. After the first COVID cases.

I've seen the manifests.

I've seen the email chains.

"Shipment cleared for transfer to WIV."
"Samples confirmed: AIV YN-14, H5N1-SC-91, H7N9 recombinant." "Maintain cold chain; forward metadata upon receipt."

Let me ask you:

If we were in the middle of the worst global outbreak in a century—
why the hell were we still shipping ***bird flu*** to a lab we were supposedly investigating?

Because we weren't investigating anything.

We were **protecting the channels**.

And when the heat was on coronaviruses? We used it.

We **camouflaged everything else behind the smoke**.

Metabiota handled logistics.

They'll tell you they were just the middleman.

Fine.

But the middleman sees **everything.**

And they kept the books.

Yunnan.
Samples collected.
Shipped to Wuhan via Shenzhen.
Documentation uploaded.
Funding logged.

Not just viruses—*live virus.

And yes, I signed off on some of the funding.

No, I don't regret it.

Because we needed to **know what was possible**.

And let me tell you:

It was possible.

What we found in those samples?

Certain strains with ***dual receptor affinity***.
They could bind to both avian and human receptors.

That's not a red flag.
That's a **biological double agent**.

And we moved those sequences around like playing cards.

Wuhan.
Hong Kong.
Zurich.

Until someone drew the wrong hand.

Now you tell me:

What's more likely?

That a once-in-a-century coronavirus jumped to humans at the exact moment we were escalating bird flu enhancements?

Or that ***something else happened first***
—and we used COVID to make you stop asking?
This was the move I made quietly.

The samples kept flowing.
The headlines didn't follow.

And when the world asked where it all began?

I gave you a virus with training wheels
to keep your eyes off the one that still has claws.

The Sample That Disappeared

Here's what we know.

Sometime between **October and December 2019**,
a sample labeled **H5N1-YZ-ß.23** was transferred from a regional
Chinese biobank to a "collaborative
U.S. partner lab."

That's the sanitized version.

The real one?

It went to **Aberdeen Proving Ground**.

U.S. Army Medical Research Institute of Infectious Diseases.

USAMRIID.

You only send a virus there for **two reasons**:

1. It's incredibly dangerous.
2. You're not allowed to admit where it came from.

Now let me tell you what's **supposed** to happen next.

You log the sample.
You sequence it.
You upload it to GenBank or GISAID with metadata: host species, collection date, passage history.

That's protocol.

That's science.

That's ***the law***.

But this sample?

Never shows up.

No sequence.
No publication.
No internal NIH citation.

It drops off the map.

Even the tracking sheet in PREDICT's cloud storage has a note:

"Processing status: withheld. Awaiting instruction."

Whose instruction?

We never asked.

Because when something gets sent to a DTRA lab and disappears?

That's **the instruction**.

I asked around.

Quietly.

No emails. No calendar invites. Just a few coffee breaks, a few favors.

What I heard?

That strain was **unusually virulent** in ferret models.
And had signs of ***prior passage***.

Which means—

It had already been enhanced.
Somewhere.
By someone.

Possibly in one of **our** labs.
Possibly in a ***partner*** lab with a looser policy on what gets logged and what gets shredded.

You think SARS-CoV-2 was scary?

H5N1-YZ-ß.23 had a ***case fatality rate north of 50% in mammals***.
Airborne.
And stable at room temperature for longer than it should've been.

I didn't see the full profile.
I didn't want to.

Because seeing it makes you **accountable** for what happens next. I asked one more question before I stopped asking entirely.

I asked:

"Was it natural?"

The guy just looked at me.

Didn't blink.
Didn't smile.
Didn't speak.

He just shook his head.

So what did we do?

We buried it.

Not literally—although that's possible.

I mean **structurally**.

We made sure that ***nothing that leaked from that sample could ever become the headline***.

Because the moment that strain gets linked to our network—PREDICT, EcoHealth, WIV, UC Davis?

It's over.

Not just my job.

Not just the NIH.

The whole house.

This is the part I don't talk about in interviews.

This is the thing I let die in the margins,
so you'd chase a pangolin in a wet market
instead of asking what else was stored in the -80°C freezer at USAMRIID.

This is the virus that didn't leak.

Because we leaked something **less dangerous** first.

Something easier to explain.

Something you could survive.

Something I could walk away from.

The Vaccine Came First

Want to know how you can tell it was all backwards?

The vaccine came first.

Not the virus.
Not the panic.
Not the spike in wastewater data.
Not the WHO emergency alert.

The contracts.

The platforms.

The ***platform rehearsals***.

DARPA called it *Prophecy*.

The premise was simple:

"Develop countermeasures before the pathogen emerges."

Sounds noble, right?

Until you realize what that means:

"Create vaccines for viruses that don't exist yet,
using data from lab-built mutations
based on models of what might go wrong."

That's not preparedness.

That's **time travel with plausible deniability**.

They were modeling H5N1 variants.
Not coronaviruses.
Not pangolins.
Not seafood stalls.

Bird flu.

In East Asia.
In ferrets.
In silico.

They even ran ***a trial batch of mRNA-based candidates*** in early 2019.
Pfizer wasn't involved yet.
But **Moderna was**.

Moderna—who'd never successfully released a product before—suddenly has ***mRNA libraries for influenza-class threats***.

Funny how that works.

Then the trials under Prophecy failed.

Why?

Because the modified H5N1 strains were too unstable.
Too hot.

They killed the ferrets too fast.
They didn't give the vaccine time to work.
And the platform couldn't adjust.

That's when DARPA wrote the internal brief:

"We need a viral class with broader public tolerance and lower lethality. Recommend pivot to seasonal coronavirus backbones."

Wait—what?

You were developing the platform for bird flu
and suddenly you ***pivot to coronaviruses***?

Before SARS-CoV-2 exists?

Yeah.
I raised an eyebrow too.

But I didn't stop it.

Because it was **easier to test mRNA in a sandbox virus** than admit the real one was too dangerous to even discuss.

Then came the ***contracts***.

Late 2019:

- **BARDA** starts "engagement conversations" with mRNA developers.
- **NIH holds an mRNA scalability workshop**.
- **CEPI starts building distribution models** based on projected pandemic timelines.

All **before the outbreak**.

Before the word ***COVID*** ever shows up in a meeting invite.

We were preparing the parachute
before we pushed anyone out of the plane.

Why?

Because the bird flu drill told us **we couldn't land it**.

We needed ***a different pathogen***
to justify ***the same solution***.

One that scared people enough to surrender,
but not enough to panic.

One that required ***new infrastructure***
but didn't ***wipe out the subjects***.

And so—

COVID.

That's the real origin story.

Not a bat.
Not a lab.
Not even me.

Just a contract,
signed before the fire started,
for a hose we didn't know how to aim.

Emergency Use Was the Product

Everyone thinks Operation Warp Speed was a miracle.

It wasn't.

It was **a salvage operation**.

Because when the *Prophecy* drills crashed,
when the avian flu platforms failed,
when the DoD realized the ferrets were dying too fast for PR to catch up—

we needed **a new narrative vehicle**.

Not a new technology.

We already had the tech.

We just didn't have the ***story***.

mRNA was sitting on a shelf.

Capped. Sequenced.
Stuck in preclinical purgatory.
Too new to approve.
Too scary to fund.
Too weird for flu.

But then—

COVID.

Suddenly all the objections vanished.

Safety data? Compressed.
Animal studies? Skipped.
Long-term effects? TBD.

The public didn't want trials.

They wanted ***relief***.

And what they got?

A technology trial disguised as humanitarian response.

Because that's what Operation Warp Speed really was:

Not a vaccine deployment.

A ***platform deployment***.

You think it was about "getting shots in arms"?

That was marketing.

What we were actually testing was:

- mRNA delivery infrastructure
- Cold chain logistics
- Regulatory bypass agility
- Public tolerance for experimental tech
- Media synchronization under pressure
- Global adoption rates by income tier

You don't need five vaccines for a single disease.

You need five data sets for the ***same product line***.

This wasn't public health.

It was ***scalable platform testing under emergency authority***.

And the emergency?

Oh, we made sure to keep it alive.

Every time the virus cooled down?

New variant.
New wave.
New metric.

Remember when deaths mattered?

Then cases mattered.
Then "hospital strain."
Then "long COVID."

Each time we moved the target,
we preserved the ***emergency***.

Because the emergency wasn't just narrative glue.

It was **legal cover**.

You can't approve an untested tech at scale unless there's **no alternative**.

That's the EUA loophole.

And we drove a ***fleet*** through it.

Hydroxychloroquine?
Destroyed.

Ivermectin?
Mocked.

Natural immunity?
Buried.

Every time a door opened that could lead ***away*** from mRNA?

We slammed it shut.

Not because the alternatives didn't work.

But because ***they made the emergency go away***.

And we couldn't afford that.

Not with the contracts signed.
Not with the platforms humming.
Not with ***billions on the table***.

If you wanted to condition an entire population to accept an experimental platform…

Would you do it during a time of peace?

Or would you do it during a ***panic***?

Exactly.

Because panic doesn't just sell urgency.

It **erases alternatives**.

We learned that from **avian flu**.

Every time we ran a simulation,
every time we printed the death projections,
every time we floated the "what-if" mutation scenarios—

we watched people shift.

They got smaller.
Quieter.
More compliant.

And most importantly?

They **started asking what they should believe**,
not what they could verify.

That's not an accident.

That's ***learned helplessness***. It works like this:

1. ***Scare them***. (High CFR, invisible enemy, exponential spread.)
2. ***Contradict yourself***. (Masks don't work / wait, yes they do.)

3. ***Shift the blame***. (It's the unvaccinated. It's misinformation.)
4. ***Offer one solution***. (Lockdowns, mandates, shots.)

Now watch what happens.

People don't rebel.

They ***comply harder***.

Because they want ***the fear to make sense***.

Avian flu gave us the model.

COVID gave us ***the scale***.

And the best part?

We built heroes and villains.

Every society needs that in a crisis.

Heroes:

- Healthcare workers (but only if vaccinated)
- Experts who agree
- Blue-check virologists
- People who "follow the science"

Villains:

- Anyone who asked a question too early
- Anyone who cited a paper we hadn't discredited yet
- Anyone who said "natural immunity" out loud

You weren't debating facts.

You were ***joining a side***.

And once you pick a side?

You'll believe anything.

As long as it means ***you were right all along***.

We didn't invent this in 2020.

We ***tested it in 2015, 2017, 2019***.

The avian flu tabletop drills all ran the same psychological loop:

- Use media to amplify fear.
- Use experts to sanctify obedience.
- Use data to confuse rather than clarify.
- Use time pressure to silence doubt.
- And above all?

Reward submission.

You didn't "trust the science."

You trusted the ***reward function***.

Applause for masking.
Likes for lockdowns.
Job protection for silence.

You were trained like a lab rat.

Same way we train viruses.

Same way we train narratives.

Same way we trained ***ourselves***.

I didn't manipulate facts.

I manipulated **how you metabolized fear**.

And once you learned to digest fear as virtue?

I never had to lie again.

You did it for me.

The Vocabulary Was Preloaded

Words matter.

We didn't need you to understand what was happening.
We just needed you to have ***a script*** in your head when it did.

We started planting it during **avian flu**.

Over years.

Through ***drills, press briefings, white papers, and softly sponsored media***.

Until suddenly, the moment we said:

"Flatten the curve."

You knew exactly what to do.

Let me give you some of our greatest hits.

"Zero COVID."

That didn't come from some monk in a PPE robe.

That came from **avian flu modeling** out of Singapore and Australia, mid-2010s.

We used it as a ***hypothetical containment strategy***—not because it worked, but because it provided a ***goal so perfect it justified permanent control***.

It was ***unreachable on purpose***.

Because chasing it gave us endless leash.

"The New Normal"

You think that was a natural evolution of language?

We tested that phrase ***in surveys during a 2017 avian flu tabletop simulation***.
It performed incredibly well among mid-career professionals and upper-middle-class urban dwellers.

Why?

Because it **promised comfort inside conformity**.

A world where if you obeyed,
you'd be safe—
but only **if everyone else did, too**.

Which gave us **social policing**.

You weren't just afraid of the virus.

You were afraid of your ***neighbor's behavior***.

That was the goal.

"Noncompliant"

That was an avian flu term.

Originally used in ***quarantine simulation memos***.

Later deployed in ***real-time media narratives*** to imply danger without legal language.

We didn't call people "criminals."
We called them "noncompliant."

Same effect.
No due process.

We made disagreement sound like ***a public health violation***.

And you thanked us for it.

"Flatten the Curve"

We invented that one **in a PowerPoint**.

Literally.

A slide from an avian flu workshop on behavioral compliance during school closures.

The original model was bullshit—assumptions on top of assumptions.

But the ***image was sticky***.

Two curves.

One tall. One flat.

You didn't care about the math.

You remembered ***the shape***.

That's not epidemiology.

That's **graphic design as psychological warfare**.

We gave you ***mnemonics of obedience***.

Phrases you could repeat.
Tweet.
Put on yard signs.
Say on Zoom calls to let people know you were **safe**.

The words didn't describe the world.

They **constructed it**.

And it worked.

It worked so well we stopped calling it messaging
and started calling it ***risk communication architecture***.

Which sounds fancy.

But really?

It's just ***branding for panic***.
I didn't invent the phrases.

I just ***slid them into your head before you needed them***.

So that when the world changed,
you'd already know how to talk about it.

And if you know how to talk about it?

You don't ask what actually happened.

We Made It Legal First

Here's something people don't get:

We didn't build the pandemic response during the pandemic.

We built it **before**.

Legally.

Because control isn't about force.
It's about ***framework***.

During the **avian flu years**—say 2005 through 2017—we weren't just experimenting with viruses.

We were experimenting with ***emergency law***.

- Model quarantine powers
- Mandatory vaccination statutes
- Liability shielding
- Isolation authority
- Cross-border data sharing
- Civil restriction thresholds

We didn't call it martial law.
We called it ***public health preparedness***.

Same thing.

Better branding.

In the wake of **H5N1**, **H7N9**, and **MERS**, the playbook was drafted:

- Federal health emergency declarations
- Emergency Use Authorizations
- State-level lockdown models
- Suspension of HIPAA for contact tracing
- Platform partnerships for "disinformation containment"

All of it was there.

Waiting.

We even wrote ***trigger language*** into state public health codes:

"Governor may take such actions as deemed necessary upon declaration of a pandemic emergency…"

"Such actions" turned out to be:

- Closing your business
- Banning your church
- Separating you from your dying parent
- Injecting your child with a vaccine that skipped animal trials
- Removing your social media account for quoting peer-reviewed science too early

And we did it all without new laws.

Because we didn't need them.

We ***built the emergency powers into the architecture***.

You think ***Warp Speed*** was fast?

The legal warp speed was ***faster***.

Because it didn't need to ask.
It just needed to be ***activated***.

Let me tell you how you know we planned it:

Because every agency, every institution, every platform—

pivoted the same week.

That's not improvisation.

That's **execution**.

Even the courts flinched.

You think judges understand viral kinetics?

No.

They saw ***emergency declarations***.

They saw ***technical language***.

They deferred.

To me.
To CDC.
To the **very structure we built to override them**.

That's how we skipped ***the Constitution***.

Not by violating it.

By ***routing around it with language we wrote in the fog of bird flu drills***.

And when we tested it under COVID?

It held.

I didn't really break the law.

I just ***built a legal maze so efficient***
you didn't realize you were already inside it.

And by the time you found the exit?

We had ***moved the fences***.

The Suppression System Was Already Built

Let's make one thing clear.

We didn't build censorship during COVID.

We **activated** it.

Like flipping a breaker in a building you didn't know had power.

The schematics were drawn during **avian flu**.

It started small:

- University policy drafts on "misinformation risk"
- WHO guidance on "pre-bunking" narratives
- DARPA-funded studies on "information contagion"
- Social contagion modeling at MIT and Stanford

At the time, we called it ***health communication resilience***.

Sounds nice.

What it meant?

Pre-authorized narrative control.

We didn't censor you because we were afraid of you.

We censored you because we had already **redefined speech as a vector**.

The minute we decided that "disinformation" was a **public health threat**, we could **treat your opinion like a virus**.

And once it's a virus?

We can isolate it.
Suppress it.
Eradicate it.
Trace its contacts.
Block its transmission.

All without ever filing a lawsuit.

This wasn't a response.

It was **pre-built enforcement**.

Let me show you how:

Platform Compliance

In 2016, during H7N9 panic cycles, the WHO floated a paper to social media executives: "Exploring cooperative frameworks for narrative containment during biological crises." Most people ignored it.

Facebook didn't.

They built ***the early trust-and-safety dashboards*** off that model.

And we thanked them with ***funding, access, and public praise***.

By 2020?

They were ***deputized***.

Contact Tracing

It didn't start with COVID.

It started with **influenza network modeling**.

We tested ***geo-fencing compliance drills*** in 2013 in response to bird flu mutation clusters in China.

They failed.

So we built better tools.

Apple and Google didn't invent contact tracing apps.

They were ***asked to make them interoperable*** long before you heard of SARS-CoV-2.

And they did.

Because they wanted to help.

And because **we knew they would**.

Vaccine Passports

The term didn't exist.

The concept did.

Modeled under "serology access protocols" in avian flu whitepapers around 2015.

Basic idea: tie movement or service access to proof of immunological status.

We ran ***simulation frameworks in coordination with DHS and IATA*** under "international travel bio-certification stress tests."

Results?

Clunky.
But viable.

COVID gave us ***the user base***.

None of this was reactive.

It was **stored protocol**.

Waiting for a **safe-enough emergency** to activate.

Bird flu was too lethal to risk public panic.

COVID?

Perfect panic-to-survival ratio.

Enough danger to scare you.
Not enough to kill the tools.

I didn't create the censorship machine.

I just ***kept it oiled until the right fire gave me a reason to run it at full speed***.

And you?

You logged in every day.
You obeyed the popups.
You reported your neighbor.
You thanked the algorithm for the silence.

That's not coercion.

That's ***compliance built upstream***.

The Real Leak Was Moral

By now, you're probably wondering:

"How could you all go along with this?" Easy.

Because ***the first leak wasn't biological***.

It was **ethical**.

It started slow.

- Run a trial without full animal data? *Okay, but only this once.*
- Skip the FOIA response window? *National security.*
- Change the definition of "gain-of-function"? *It's complicated.*
- Exclude contradictory evidence from public briefings? *Too early to confuse people.*

Each step felt small.
Justified.
Necessary.

But what we were really doing?

Training ourselves to treat honesty like a luxury.

And once we crossed that line?

It didn't feel like a line anymore.

It felt like ***policy***.

The real pandemic wasn't the virus.

It was the moment we decided **you couldn't handle the truth**.

That your job was to comply,
not comprehend.

We called it:

- "Public trust management"
- "Health communication"
- "Narrative alignment"

But really?

It was ***gaslighting with citations***.

We knew the masks didn't work the way we said.
We knew the trials were rushed.
We knew the data was contradictory.
We knew the tools were coercive.
We knew the messaging was manipulative.
We knew the platforms were political.
We knew the press was performing.

And we did it anyway.

Because ***fear is useful.***

And once the public's afraid?

You can do almost anything to them—

as long as you call it care.

That was the real leak:

The normalization of control.

We didn't hide it.

We didn't need to.

You called it ***the new normal.***

You **asked** us to keep going.

To mandate your neighbors.
To restrict the unclean.
To fire the disobedient.

To unfriend the curious.
To silence the skeptics.

You did it with pride.
With hashtags.

Because we gave you the story.

And you liked your part in it.

I didn't corrupt the system.

I just ***let it show its true face***.

And the mask?

Was never for the virus.

It was for ***you***.

What the Silence Covered

You've seen the COVID timeline.

You've memorized it.

- December 2019: cluster in Wuhan.
- January 2020: genome release.
- February: lockdowns begin.
- March: pandemic declared.
- April: masks.
- May: George Floyd.
- June: "the science is evolving."

It's the most **publicized biological event in human history**.

But you know what's weird?

In that same window,
the avian flu timeline stops.

Flatline.

Gone.

We had ***over a decade*** of routine surveillance:

- Monthly WHO FluNet updates.
- National Institute bulletins.
- Genetic sequences uploaded to GISAID.
- Outbreak reports in poultry populations.
- Lab studies on recombination and vaccine drift.

And then?

Silence.

Right when it should've been screaming.

You know what we should've seen in Q4 2019?

- Ongoing sample sequences from Yunnan.
- Updates on the serial passaging studies in Guangdong.
- Military lab feedback loops from the DoD.
- Vaccine candidate reports on modified H5N1 and H7N9 strains.
- Any mention of H5N1-YZ-ß.23, the sample we quietly shelved.

Instead?

- Empty dashboards.
- Dead links.
- Redacted paragraphs.
- "Administrative archiving."
- "Database restructuring."

We didn't lose the data.

We buried it.

And we built ***COVID noise on top of it***.

That's how you hide a timeline:

You create a louder one.

You think COVID was about response?

COVID was ***a cover event***.

A biological smokescreen big enough to **wrap the world in narrative armor**, so no one would ask why:

- Metabiota was still routing bird flu samples into WIV in November 2019
- DARPA was running parallel vaccine drills for H5N1 the same month
- USAMRIID received a never-logged, ferret-lethal strain in early December
- CDC China staff reported "pneumonia of unknown origin" weeks before COVID was named—but ***didn't say what virus they suspected***

Want to know what it looked like?

Not panic.

Not even concern.

It looked like ***coordination***.

Of silence.

That's how you know the truth wasn't just dangerous.

It was **agreed upon**.

To be deleted.
This is the part I never had to explain.

Because ***COVID explained it for me***.

It gave you fear.
It gave you heroes.
It gave you headlines.

It gave you **enough noise to forget the missing pages**.

And that's all we needed.

CHAPTER 21

The Ritual

The Consent Ritual: Why We Told You Everything and You Still Said Yes

There's a rule.
Not a written one.
Not legal. Not constitutional.

Older than all that.

You can't trick people into walking off a cliff.
Not unless you **put up a sign first**.

You have to **warn them**.
Show them the truth.
Even if it's buried in jargon, or framed upside-down, or hidden in the footnotes.

Because if they see it and **go along anyway**— that's not harm. That's **consent**.

You want to know why we told you masks work, then didn't, then did again?

You want to know why we changed definitions midstream, right on the CDC website?

Why we published the *DEFUSE* proposal in the open literature?
Why we bragged about furin cleavage sites?
Why Peter Daszak said in 2016 that pandemic profits would rise "if we do it right"?

Because we **had to**.

We had to give you the data.
The proof.
The logic.

But we also had to deliver it in a way that made you **ignore it**.

That's the game.

The ritual goes like this:

1. **Reveal the plan**—in some dry government memo, a boring white paper, or a scientific preprint with 37 co-authors.
2. **Wrap it in credibility**—peer review, institutional logos, words like "robust" and "meta-analysis."
3. **Contradict it in public**—have a trusted face (like me) and say something that **sounds** confident but doesn't match the data.
4. **Let you decide** what to believe.

And when you choose the contradiction over the content?

That's **your signature on the contract**.

You think we lied?
No.

We gave you the truth.

We **hid it in plain sight**.

- We told you the vaccine trials never tested for transmission.
- We told you the risk for kids was statistically negligible.
- We told you about the lab partnerships, the gain-of-function loopholes, the spike protein mutations.

You just didn't want that to be the story.

You wanted hope.
You wanted order.
You wanted safety wrapped in a surgical mask and served with a booster every fall.

We gave you what you asked for.

And you thanked us.

There's an ancient principle behind all this.
Call it karma, call it natural law, call it *the big guy upstairs*.

You can't enslave people.
But you can **convince them to put the chains on themselves**.

And the way you do that?

You tell them **exactly what you're doing**,
but deliver it in a form they're trained to **ignore**.

You say, "This isn't about control."
You say, "We're here to help."
You say, "This is science."

And the moment they nod—
You're free to proceed.

Because **they chose it**.

You think DEFUSE was a smoking gun?

It was a **permission slip**.

We published it.
We cited it.
We put it in the NIH grant database, right next to the bat coronavirus serial passaging experiments.

And no one stopped us.

That means the rules were followed.

Whatever I did, I did it according to **the law behind the law**.
The one that says you have to show your hand—
but not **highlight** the cards.

And if you let me deal anyway?

That's not deception.

That's agreement.

The Magic Trick: How We Made You Thank Us for the Fire

Every good con has a tell.
Ours was kindness.
Concern.
Reassurance.

We weren't selling compliance—we were selling **salvation**.
And once you believe you're being saved,
you'll set yourself on fire if we tell you it's for the greater good.

The trick was simple:

1. **Start the fire.**
   Maybe it's a virus. Maybe it's fear. Maybe it's both.
2. **Promise a solution.**
   A lockdown. A mandate. A miracle mRNA shot with the **"safest profile in vaccine history"**—developed in ten months.
3. **Deliver the solution with conditions.**
   We don't make you take it. But try flying, working, or buying groceries without it.
4. **Then let you believe it was your idea.**

If we did it right—and we did—you'd light the match, breathe in the smoke, and then **thank us** for keeping the room warm.

The trick works because we made you part of it.

We turned science into religion:

- *Peer-reviewed gospels*
- *Experts as clergy*
- *Dissent as heresy*
- *Censorship as hygiene*

Then we gave you rituals.
Hand sanitizer.
Elbow bumps.
Six feet of holy distance.

We wrapped it all in **moral obligation**.
You weren't just protecting yourself.
You were saving **Grandma**.

You weren't masking because we told you to.
You were **a good person**.

That's how it works.
You don't force the subject to take the deal.
You make them **feel righteous for accepting i**t.

Look at the vaccine campaign:

We told you it would stop the virus.
Then we told you it would stop you from dying.
Then we told you it would stop severe illness.
Then we told you to get it anyway.

Every step down the ladder,
we reworded the script so you wouldn't notice we'd already hit the ground.

And you didn't rebel.
You **applauded**.
You took selfies.
You scolded your neighbors.
You posted your card like it was a medal.

That's not science.
That's sorcery.

And the spell?

You cast it on yourself.

Why did we tell you so much and hide so little?

Because we didn't have to hide it.
We just had to **surround it** with noise.
With celebrity endorsements.
With blue banners on social media.
With "fact-checks" that never addressed the actual claim.

We didn't need to erase the evidence.
We just needed to **make the truth feel inconvenient**.

And once you're uncomfortable,
you'll reach for whatever story fits your fear.

We provided that story.

You paid with belief.

I didn't lie.
I performed.

And you weren't the audience.
You were the **volunteer**.

You got on stage.
You helped me misdirect.
You clapped before the reveal.

And when I made your agency disappear?

You helped.

Because that's how the trick works.

Every. Single. Time.

Your Silence Was the Signature

I used to think consent required action.

A signature.
A vote.
An opt-in.

But that's not how real systems work.
Not the ones that matter.

In real systems, **silence is enough**.
Looking away is **permission**.
Not asking questions is **agreement**.

And in 2020, you didn't sign a form.

You **let it happen**.

When we locked down the schools?

You told yourselves it was temporary.
That we were "flattening the curve."
That we'd reassess after two weeks.

You knew.
You saw the data.
You watched your kids fall behind.
You watched toddlers try to learn language behind cloth.

But you didn't push back.

Not really.
You made excuses.
You forwarded articles.
You waited for someone else to object first.

No one did.

So we kept going.

When we told you the vaccine didn't stop infection—but required a mandate anyway?

You grumbled.
You rationalized.
You updated your LinkedIn with a little syringe emoji.

That wasn't resistance.
That was **absorption**.

You **absorbed the lie**, because the alternative was harder.
It meant confronting the reality that maybe, just maybe, the people in charge were using your goodwill against you.

And nobody wants to be that guy at the dinner party.

So you stayed quiet.

And the machine heard that silence.

It translated it as **yes**.

We didn't need to censor you.
You censored yourselves.

You self-edited.
You whispered.
You said, "Well, I'm not an expert, but…"

We taught you that **only experts get to speak**.
Then we made sure all the experts said the same thing.

That wasn't science.
That was **choreography**.

And you let it play.

You think the contract was verbal?
Or written?

No.

The contract was **in your compliance**.

- You wore the mask even when no one watched.
- You kept your distance in the park.
- You got the booster—even when it didn't make sense—because it was "the right thing to do."

That wasn't safety.
That was **a signature in behavior**.

A way of saying:
"I agree to the terms. Even if I don't understand them."

I didn't do it *to* you.
I did it **with your permission**.

You didn't scream.
You didn't resist.
You didn't walk out of the theater.

You sat there.
You watched.
And when the credits rolled?

You clapped.

CHAPTER 22

And Then the Curtain Drops

Let's say the play is over.

The lights dim.
The banners come down.
The slogans fade.
The fact-checkers unplug their servers.
The dashboards stop updating.

It's quiet now.

And I step out from behind the scrim.

No cameras.
No microphones.
No White House briefing room.
Just me.
And you.
And the truth that was always there, flickering behind the projection.

You want me to confess?

Fine.

We made a show of science.
We built a morality play out of policy.
We engineered consent with panic, and called it "public trust."

We were architects of uncertainty and curators of obedience.
We took your fear and offered theater.
And you bought tickets. Every time.

We broke things we never repaired.
We forced choices we never faced ourselves.
We said "we're in this together" from the safety of private jets and green rooms.

And in the end, we called it a success.

Not because it was.
But because **you were still applauding**.

And yet—

There's one rule we couldn't break.

Not even with all the funding, the labs, the models, the media.

The rule is this:

You can't harm someone unless they accept it.

It's old.
Older than bioethics.
Older than the WHO.
Older than virology.

It's woven into the wiring of the world.

The cosmic contract.
The divine non-disclosure.

So we told you.
Over and over.
In fine print.
In conference panels.
In op-eds and acronyms and dry academic language.

We laid it at your feet.
And waited for you to say,
"*That sounds good to me.*"

And you did.

You accepted the terms.

And once you do that—

Well, we're allowed to proceed.

Now the curtain falls.

Not with justice.
Not with a tribunal.
Not with a bang.

But with understanding.
Or maybe just the echo of it.

Everything I did
was because I was permitted.
Because I was *believed.*
Because I was needed.

Because you asked for someone to save you.

And I raised my hand.

So here we are.

You're standing in the ashes.
And I'm walking off the stage.

The mask is gone.
The suit is hung.
The voice is quiet.

And somewhere, behind all this,
a projector is still humming.

Still playing the story.

Even though
you already know
how it ends.

Appendix

The Diary of Anthony Fauci

2019

OCTOBER 18 · FRIDAY

EVIDENCE
CASE# AF1521
ITEM# 67
INITIALS GT

Event 201, NYC
They say it's a tabletop exercise.
But it's more like a read-through.
Johns Hopkins, Gates, WEF— lots of people using the word "resilience."
Scenario? Coronavirus, zoonotic, jumps in a food market, destabilizes global supply chains.
We spend two hours workshopping how to crush "disinformation."
We spend zero time on how to contain a virus—it's all about how to contain the public reaction.
No mention of Wuhan.
But the framework is all there.
Censorship coordination.
Unified messaging.
Trusted messengers.

Nobody asks why this exercise appeared now.
I already know.

CONFIRMATION:

EVIDENCE
CASE# AF1521
ITEM# 69
INITIALS GT

2019
NOVEMBER 1 · FRIDAY

Bethesda.

Rumors from the PREDICT network.
Yunnan team collected a new strain
in October—"concerning binding
behavior."
Daszak has the sequence. WIV has
the sample.

No one at UC Davis saying anything.
Metabiota's logs show cold-chain transfer
to Wuhan completed on Oct 27.

We sent them the firewood.
We sent them the match.
Now I'm watching for smoke.

CONFIRMATION:

2019
NOVEMBER 12 · TUESDAY

EVIDENCE
CASE# AF1521
ITEM# 71
INITIALS GT

Off book meeting, DTRA liaison.

DARPA's tracking movement
around WIV.
Low-level chatter flagged by intel:
"dead researchers," "internal
lockdown," "respiratory failure."

I ask if we have any sequence data.
He says we had it—and then <u>EcoHealth
pulled the plug</u>.

Daszak is suddenly very interested in
WHO press strategy.

I don't say it out loud, but
<u>it's already out</u>.

CONFIRMATION:

2019
DECEMBER 30 · MONDAY

EVIDENCE
CASE# AF1521
ITEM# 72
INITIALS GT

Genomic data scrubbed from online repositories by Chinese.
CDC looped in.
No comment.

Daszak already drafting a statement about "conspiracies."

Andersen is pinging Slack groups.
I get my first email from NASEM asking how we want to "frame" the response.

They haven't named the virus yet.

But we're already workshopping the story.

CONFIRMATION:

2020

JANUARY 6 · MONDAY

EVIDENCE
CASE# AF1521
ITEM# 74
INITIALS GT

We're past the quiet stage.

I advise internal teams to begin containment—<u>not of the virus, but of the discourse</u>.

We don't need answers yet.

We need <u>unity</u>.

EVIDENCE
CASE # AF1521
ITEM # 76
INITIALS GT

2020
JANUARY 9 · THURSDAY

Peter's drafting the first talking points.
Good.
He understands tempo.

Key phrases:
– "Natural origin highly likely"
– "No credible lab link"
– "Stop misinformation before it spreads"

We don't need to prove anything.
We just need to define what's credible.

EVIDENCE
CASE# AF1521
ITEM# 77
INITIALS GT

2020
JANUARY 15 · WEDNESDAY

State wants to mention a lab accident.

We need that door closed.

Before the public even knows there's a <u>door</u> there.

They cut the reference.

Correct move.

EVIDENCE
CASE# AF1521
ITEM# 79
INITIALS GT

2020

FEBRUARY 1 · SATURDAY

War Council Zoom call: Andersen, Garry, Holmes, Baric.

I convene. I listen.

They say what I already know:
"The spike looks engineered."
"The furin site doesn't belong."

We discuss scenarios. Then I bring them back to reality:
"You don't publish evidence—we publish confidence."

They nod.

Within 48 hours, the draft of Proximal Origin is under way.

CONFIRMATION:

2020
FEBRUARY 10 · MONDAY

EVIDENCE
CASE# AF1521
ITEM# 81
INITIALS GT

Starting on feb 4, we worked
up messaging:

Private uncertainty becomes public
certainty.

We remove phrases like:
- "Unusual features"
- "Unlikely recombination path"

And replace them with:
- "Consistent with evolution"
- "No lab origin evidence"

I don't edit directly.
I suggest shape.

Baric knows the rhythm.
Andersen delivers the syntax.

By the time the paper's ready, the
story is locked.

EVIDENCE
CASE# AF1521
ITEM# 83
INITIALS GT

2020
FEBRUARY 11 · TUESDAY

Realignment:

Face-to-face with Bavic.
"Do you believe it?"

He smiles. Doesn't answer.
He knows the answer doesn't matter.

What matters is containment—
of questions, of liability.

CONFIRMATION:

EVIDENCE
CASE# AF1521
ITEM# 85
INITIALS GT

2020
FEBRUARY 19 · WEDNESDAY

The Lancet Letter deploys.

Peter executes beautifully.

Twenty-seven scientists.
No disclosures.
No dissent.

It lands like scripture.

Suddenly, lab leak isn't a theory—
it's a threat to science itself.
Now, anyone who asks the right
question becomes part of the wrong
team.

How you pre-empt a scandal:
You define the limits of acceptable
thought before the facts catch up.

CONFIRMATION:

2020

MARCH 2 · MONDAY

EVIDENCE
CASE# AF1521
ITEM# 87
INITIALS GT

Memo to HHS.

We push messaging directive to focus public attention on mitigation.

Avoid origin debates,
Promote consensus
We didn't hide the truth.

We <u>smothered it in structure.</u>

EVIDENCE
CASE# AF1521
ITEM# 88
INITIALS GT

2020
APRIL 3 · FRIDAY

Mask Directive. We change the guidance.

Not because the data changed—because the optics did.

Public needs a ritual. A signal.
They can't see aerosols.
They can wrap cloth around their faces and be good people.

Push compliance now. Justify it later.

2020

APRIL 28 · TUESDAY

EVIDENCE
CASE# AF1521
ITEM# 89
INITIALS GT

Daszak emails leak.

We built this house together.
Now we're boarding up
the windows—
from the inside.

I don't respond.
He's panicking.
I need him calm.
We need his name on the defense,
not the confession.

CONFIRMATION:

2020

MAY 12 · TUESDAY

EVIDENCE
CASE# AF1521
ITEM# 91
INITIALS GT

Senate hearing. Under Oath.
Rand Paul asks the question.
I answer carefully. I was ready.

"We did not find gain-of-function
research at the Wuhan Institute
of Virology."

That's technically true—by
our definition.
We changed the definition after the
work was done.

Nobody notices.
Headlines carry my quote
without context.

I win this round.

CONFIRMATION:

2020

MAY 20 · WEDNESDAY

EVIDENCE
CASE# AF1521
ITEM# 92
INITIALS GT

Back-channel contact from NASEM and Science editorial staff.
They ask if we want "preemptive reinforcement" of natural origin claims in upcoming coverage.

I tell them:
Early June. Pre-summer lull. Call it settled science. They agree.

This is what institutional momentum looks like.

Not conspiracy.
Convergence.

CONFIRMATION:

EVIDENCE
CASE# AF1521
ITEM# 94
INITIALS GT

2020
JUNE 15 · MONDAY

If they piece together the shipment logs, the sequence data, the Slack threads—

Then I'm not testifying.

I'm negotiating.

I keep moving.

Always forward.
Never revisit.
Never reflect.

That's how you survive a leak:
You get ahead of the inquiry before the questions arrive.

EVIDENCE
CASE# AF1521
ITEM# 95
INITIALS GT

2020
JULY 7 · THURSDAY

Operation Warp Speed is moving fast.
Efficacy must mean protection from symptoms, not preventing infection.
Otherwise, the data will betray us by winter.

Science is about precision.

Messaging: controlled imprecision.

2020

AUGUST 14 · FRIDAY

EVIDENCE
CASE# AF1521
ITEM# 96
INITIALS GT

Moderna wants my quote for press release.

I give them something neutral: "An important milestone in the race to end the pandemic."

What I don't say:
Was never tested
for transmission.
Never tracked long-term effects.
We just needed a product.

2020

AUGUST 28 · FRIDAY

EVIDENCE
CASE# AF1521
ITEM# 98
INITIALS GT

Someone flags a preprint modeling the spike protein as "evolutionarily unlikely."
I forward to Daszak.

He replies:
"I'll handle it."

He always does.
He understands the difference between science and story.

One finds the truth.
The other survives it.

CONFIRMATION:

2020

SEPTEMBER 6 · SUNDAY

EVIDENCE
CASE# AF1521
ITEM# 100
INITIALS GT

They're writing profiles now.

The Atlantic does well for me.
I will pay them back well.

"Fauci as America's Dad."
"Fauci: The Reluctant Hero."
"Trust in Science Rests on One
Man's Shoulders."

Good.

Hero status isn't a media move.
It's a liability shield.

I lean in.
Slow nods.
Measured cadence.
White coat, no tie.

CONFIRMATION:

EVIDENCE
CASE# AF1521
ITEM# 101
INITIALS GT

2020
NOVEMBER 3 · TUESDAY

I stay out of view.

I've become too visible.

To half the country, I'm the only adult in the room.

To the other half, I'm Mengele in a white coat.

Both are wrong.
But both are useful.

Either way, they'll need me on the other side.

2020

DECEMBER 2 · WEDNESDAY

EVIDENCE
CASE# AF1521
ITEM# 103
INITIALS GT

We finalize EUA positioning.

Downplay lack of transmission data

Emphasize risk to the unvaccinated.

If we make vaccination a moral obligation, we don't need to prove it works for health.

We just need compliance.

2021

JANUARY 6 · WEDNESDAY

Capitol distraction is
Perfect timing.

All attention is elsewhere.
We post a quiet CDC memo:

"Vaccinated individuals may still
transmit the virus."
No press conference.
No tweet.

We never said the vaccines stop
spread.
But we let people believe it.
Now we start dialing it back.

Gently.

2021

JANUARY 20 · WEDNESDAY

EVIDENCE
CASE# AF1521
ITEM# 107
INITIALS GT

–Inauguration Day–

Transfer complete.

No sudden shifts.
We make it look like continuity.

I brief Ron Klain personally.
He nods a lot. Doesn't take notes.
Good. That's how this works now.

The Biden team will own the
mandates. The passports.
The next booster wave.

I gave them the first two acts.

They'll improvise the ending.

2021
FEBRUARY 23 · TUESDAY

Drafting long-term vaccine
schedule language.
Booster timelines.
"Annual protection."

This isn't a sprint.

It's a <u>subscription model</u>.

2021

APRIL 2 · FRIDAY

EVIDENCE
CASE# AF1521
ITEM# 110
INITIALS GT

Internal memo from Israeli data analysts.

Preliminary numbers suggest natural immunity may be stronger than mRNA-induced immunity.

Bad news.

Not for science—for narrative.

If prior infection is more effective than the vaccine, then:

- Mandates become ethically fragile
- Boosters hard to sell
- EUA justification erodes

We classify the new data as "inconclusive."

Delay. Deflect.

Request more data, then sit on the request.

Buy time. Always buy time.

CONFIRMATION:

2021
APRIL 19 · MONDAY

Bret Weinstein.
Pierre Kory.
Malone.

A new front opens:
Academics who can't be dismissed
as quacks
—but refuse to fall in line.

They're saying too much:
"The trials were incomplete."
"Adverse events are underreported."
"This isn't science—it's marketing."

We label it "misinformation."
Push for deplatforming.
Tell tech companies:
"This could cost lives."
What we really mean is:
"This could cost <u>control</u>."

EVIDENCE
CASE# AF1521
ITEM# 115
INITIALS GT

2021
MAY 1 · SATURDAY

A vaccinated staff member gets infected.
Mild case. No hospitalization. But viral load is measurable.

We notify CDC. Quietly.
CDC drafts a guidance update, but doesn't publish it.

"We're still evaluating."
What we're really doing is figuring out how to say it without saying it.
People can still catch it.
They can still spread it.
But if the public hears that, we lose.
So we call them Breakthrough Cases.

"Breakthroughs are rare. Expected.
Nothing to worry about."

That works. For now.

CONFIRMATION:

2021

MAY 24 · MONDAY

EVIDENCE
CASE# AF1521
ITEM# 116
INITIALS GT

FOIA Alert. Buzz around my emails growing.

Someone found the Feb 1 Zoom call. Andersen's original statement:

"Looks engineered. Not consistent with natural evolution."

We spin it as "early confusion."
Call it "the scientific process."

We say:
"The record shows how we came to consensus."

We don't say:
"We buried what we believed."

CONFIRMATION:

EVIDENCE
CASE# AF1521
ITEM# 119
INITIALS GT

2021
JUNE 3 · THURSDAY

Someone leaks the internal EcoHealth correspondence. Vanity Fair very disappointing. What happened to them?

PREDICT timelines.
DEFUSE proposal.

Suddenly, people are using words like:
– "Cover-up"
– "Dual-use"
– "Bioweapon research"

We respond with the usual:
"No direct funding."
"Nothing we approved met the definition." "Senator Paul is misinformed."

Keep the language clean.
Keep the deniability intact.

CONFIRMATION:

2021
JUN 30 · WEDNESDAY

EVIDENCE
CASE# AF1521
ITEM# 121
INITIALS GT

If they connect the sequences to
the samples—
If they follow the money trail through UC
Davis and back to the cold storage—
If the internal Slack messages leak—

Then it's not about miscommunication
anymore.

It's about accountability.

And I don't survive that version of
the story.

So I stay visible.
I smile.
I say:

"We followed the science."

CONFIRMATION:

EVIDENCE
CASE# AF1521
ITEM# 123
INITIALS GT

2021
AUGUST 9 · MONDAY

CNN interview goes perfect, as they do.

I say:
"We're seeing waning immunity."

I don't say:
"We saw that coming in February."

I say:
"We may need additional protection."

I don't say:
"Pfizer's already booked the contracts."

They feed me the script,
I translate it into <u>reassuring authority</u>.

EVIDENCE
CASE# AF1521
ITEM# 125
INITIALS GT

2021
AUGUST 25 · WEDNESDAY

Polling shows decline in public trust.
The trend is downward.

We Didn't Lose the Science—We Lost the Silence.
Biggest drivers:
- Mask reversals
- Vaccine transmission confusion
- Suppressed early treatment questions

Natural immunity being ignored.
I remind my team:
"History is what survives scrutiny. Not what happened."
I say:
"We don't need to win everyone back. We just need to maintain majority inertia."

Momentum is the new credibility.

2021

OCTOBER 4 · MONDAY

EVIDENCE
CASE# AF1521
ITEM# 127
INITIALS GT

CDC briefing on South African Variant

B.1.1.529. Omicron.

Too many mutations to spin as incremental.
Too fast to pretend we're ahead of it.

Emergency response call with Pfizer.

I ask:
"Can you pivot the booster messaging in 10 days?"

They say:
"We already started."

Gotta love 'em

EVIDENCE
CASE# AF1521
ITEM# 128
INITIALS GT

2021
OCTOBER 15 · FRIDAY

Pivot the message.

CDC revises language:
"Up to date" replaces
"fully vaccinated."
"Booster protection" becomes
"baseline immunity."

We shift from two shots to
indefinite eligibility.

Carefully, incrementally.

Boiled frog logic.

Nobody notices.

CONFIRMATION:

2022

JANUARY 6 · THURSDAY

EVIDENCE
CASE# AF1521
ITEM# 131
INITIALS GT

Omicron is now the pandemic.

Hospitalizations dropping.
Deaths stable.
Natural immunity exploding.

The threat is over.
But the structure remains.

That was always the point.

We don't dismantle the surveillance.
We *shift its justification*.

From pandemic to "public safety."

The system doesn't need the emergency.
It needs *the precedent*.

2022

JANUARY 18 · TUESDAY

Senate hearing – Paul again. He's quoting my emails now.
He has some receipts—Andersen, Basic, early Feb calls.

I keep it calm:

"Senator, you are distorting the truth."

2022

FEBRUARY 4 · FRIDAY

EVIDENCE
CASE# AF1521
ITEM# 136
INITIALS GT

CDC drops a bomb:
"Prior infection provides strong protection—sometimes stronger than two-dose mRNA."

We don't do a press release.
No cable interviews.

We let the truth arrive silently. And nobody hears it.

Soon, it'll be harmless history.

CONFIRMATION:

2022
MAY 5 · THURSDAY

Most of the players are in position:

–Baric: quiet, protected.

–Andersen: recanted his recantation, safe.

–Daszak: burned but still salaried.

–UC Davis: never even looked at.

WIV: untouchable.

2022

JUNE 30 · THURSDAY

EVIDENCE
CASE# AF1521
ITEM# 140
INITIALS GT

The virus is over, but every system we built remains:

–Censorship infrastructure

–Emergency legal frameworks

–Biodefense budget escalators

2022
JULY 5 · TUESDAY

We finalized language:
"Dr. Fauci to step down in December after more than five decades of service."

Key word is service.
Not power.
Not control.

Service. Public service.

The press eats it up.
I give them a quote about "beginning the next chapter."

But I've already written the ending.

EVIDENCE
CASE# AF1521
ITEM# 144
INITIALS GT

2022
OCTOBER 19 · WEDNESDAY

They want me to testify one last time.

I agree—on my terms.

Closed door.
No cameras.
No curveballs.

The deal is simple:
I give you closure.
You give me exit velocity.

It works.

They shake my hand.

They let me go.

2022
NOVEMBER 3 · THURSDAY

Final White House briefing.

I tell the press:
"I'll miss this podium."

That really is the part I'll miss.

2022

DECEMBER 20 · TUESDAY

EVIDENCE
CASE# AF1521
ITEM# 149
INITIALS GT

I leave quietly.

No farewell tour.

The reporters want a quote.

"I did what I thought was right—every day."

True.

Because it was right to survive. It's always right to survive.

Always right to manage perception.
Always right to manage the ending.